QUICK AND EASY
LOW-CARB
SNACKS

Quarto.com

© 2024 Quarto Publishing Group USA Inc.
Text © 2014 Quarto Publishing Group USA Inc. and © 2016 Martina Slajerova

First Published in 2024 by New Shoe Press, an imprint of The Quarto Group,
100 Cummings Center, Suite 265-D, Beverly, MA 01915, USA.
T (978) 282-9590 F (978) 283-2742

Essential, In-Demand Topics, Four-Color Design, Affordable Price
New Shoe Press publishes affordable, beautifully designed books covering evergreen, in-demand subjects. With a goal to inform and inspire readers' everyday hobbies, from cooking and gardening to wellness and health to art and crafts, New Shoe titles offer the ultimate library of purposeful, how-to guidance aimed at meeting the unique needs of each reader. Reimagined and redesigned from Quarto's best-selling backlist, New Shoe books provide practical knowledge and opportunities for all DIY enthusiasts to enrich and enjoy their lives.

Visit Quarto.com/New-Shoe-Press for a complete listing of the New Shoe Press books.

New Shoe Press titles are also available at discount for retail, wholesale, promotional, and bulk purchase. For details, contact the Special Sales Manager by email at specialsales@quarto.com or by mail at The Quarto Group, Attn: Special Sales Manager, 100 Cummings Center, Suite 265-D, Beverly, MA 01915, USA.

10 9 8 7 6 5 4 3 2 1

ISBN: 978-0-7603-9044-3
eISBN: 978-0-7603-9045-0

The content that appears in this book previously appeared in the following books published by Fair Winds Press: *Super Low-Carb Snacks* (2019); *200 Low-Carb, High-Fat Recipes* (2014), by Dana Carpender; *Super Paleo Snacks* (2014), by Landria Voigt; *Sweet and Savory Fat Bombs* (2016), by Martina Slajerova

Library of Congress Cataloging-in-Publication Data available

Photography: Martina Slajerova and Landria Voigt

Printed in China

The information in this book is for educational purposes only. It is not intended to replace the advice of a physician or medical practitioner. Please see your health-care provider before beginning any new health program.

QUICK AND EASY
LOW-CARB
SNACKS

75 Delicious KETO and PALEO Treats for Fat Burning and Great Nutrition

MARTINA SLAJEROVA,
LANDRIA VOIGT, C.H.H.C.,
AND DANA CARPENDER

NEW SHOE PRESS

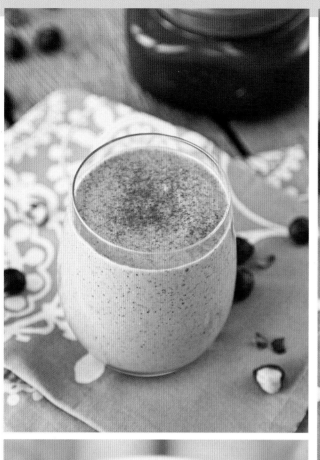

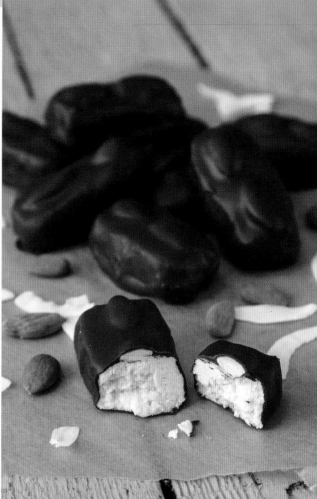

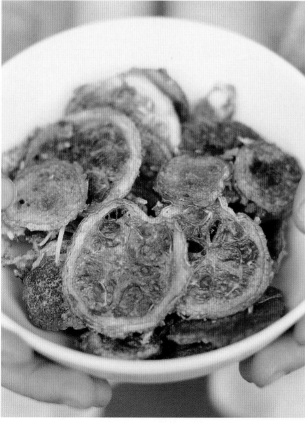

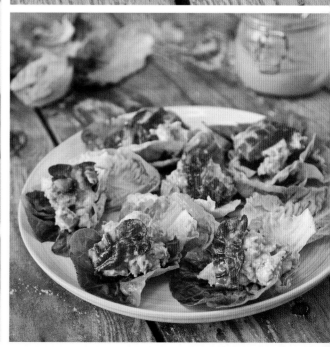

Contents

Introduction: The Importance of Healthy Snacking   6

1 The Basics:
Versatile, Homemade Nut Butters and Sugar-Free Chocolates   8

2 School and Work Snacks:
Nourishing Noshes to Fuel Your Day   28

3 At-Home Snacks:
Skip the Chips for Delicious, Healthy Options   50

4 On-the-go Snacks:
Fun and Convenient for Commutes, Carpools,
and Road Trips   70

5 Sippable Snacks:
Blissful Beverages for Any Time of Day   90

6 Safe Snacking:
Nut-Free, Dairy-Free, and Egg-Free Options   110

About the Authors   139

Index   141

Introduction

The Importance of Healthy Snacking

Almost everyone snacks. A 2010 study in the *Journal of Nutrition* found that 24 percent—nearly a quarter—of our total energy intake comes from snacks. For something that contributes to our diet as much as breakfast, lunch, and dinner do, it's somewhat surprising that relatively few people know whether they follow good snacking habits—or even that there is such a thing as a "good snack habit."

Most snacks consumed today skew toward the prepackaged and processed kinds that are high in refined sugar, white flour, gluten, and food coloring while being low in nutrition. Consuming these foods is, in general, bad for you and your health.

This book offers healthy alternatives: one-hundred low-carb, Paleo- and Keto-friendly, whole-food snacks. These snacks will satisfy your between-meals hunger and provide you with the energy you need, whether it's at work or school, on the road, at home, during a workout, or any time. They include:

"Fat bombs"—high in fat and low in protein and carbohydrates, they're the ideal snacks if you're eating low carb. Choose a fat bomb anytime, such as when you don't have time to cook and need a quick hit of energy or as pre- or post-workout snacks instead of "regular" snacks that are high in carbs.

Basic nut and seed butters and sugar-free chocolates provide the foundation for healthy snacking. Easy to make, use them in place of peanut butter, in smoothies, as a healthy way to satisfy a sweet tooth, and as the basis for other low-carb recipes.

Sippable snacks, both hot and cold, are easy to take on the go or enjoyed slowly when you have time to yourself. (Some of these recipes are high in calories, so if calories are important to you, take note and adjust accordingly.)

An entire chapter devoted to nut-free, dairy-free, and egg-free options in one easy-to-find place. (Note that additional allergy-free recipes can be found throughout the book as denoted by the icons in the "Got Allergens" chart below.)

The Benefits of Snacking

It is important to understand that snacking is not only normal, but it is also an absolutely healthy endeavor, as long as the nutritional value of the snack is beneficial. We snack for many reasons, the primary of which is to stave off hunger in between meals.

Got Allergies
If you're concerned about allergens, look for these icons at the top of recipes:

 Dairy-Free

 Egg-Free

 Nut-Free

Yet snacking provides a number of physical and cognitive perks, too. It can boost cognitive focus throughout the work and school day by helping us maintain blood sugar levels. Our bodies digest whole foods that include fats, proteins, and fiber—such as the ones in this book—at a slower and more consistent rate, and therefore release a steadier stream of glucose to the brain. Conversely, a snack that is high in refined sugar and white flour will spike insulin levels and cause one to be hungrier and less focused in a shorter time. The snacks in this book contain ingredients such as meat, eggs, and nuts that will hold hunger at bay while keeping you tack sharp.

Another benefit of snacking is that it helps prevent overeating at mealtime. There's a difference between "ruining your dinner" and preparing your body with vital nutrients. Sitting down to dinner with that "I'm famished" feeling can lead you to consume more calories than you actually need. In a state of heightened hunger, you tend to eat faster. Numerous studies have shown that individuals who eat slower typically consume fewer calories than their fast-eating peers. Science suggests this is because of a communication lag between the receptors in your stomach and those in your brain—in other words, between having a full stomach and the realization that you're satiated. So by helping quell the feeling of hunger through more consistent engagement of stomach receptors, appropriate pre-meal snacks might actually help you lose weight.

For anyone who works out or plays a sport, preworkout snacks are imperative to optimizing performance. The right balance of protein can help us keep our mind focused and increase endurance by slowing muscle breakdown during activity. Also important is having the right postworkout snacks in your bag. We lose many minerals through the excretion of sweat during exercise, and those minerals need to be replaced quickly so our bodies can work efficiently. With a deficiency of certain minerals, such as magnesium, we may have fatigue, muscle cramps, trouble maintaining blood sugar levels, and a harder time getting oxygen into our muscle cells.

Recognizing When It's Truly Time for a Snack

When you really think about it, what is it to "feel hungry"? The signs are usually much more subtle than a rumbling tummy, which can often be quelled by a glass of water, as many times we mistake thirst for hunger. Is your energy starting to wane? Perhaps your ability to focus on the task at hand is becoming more of a challenge. Are you becoming a bit more irritable? When any of these symptoms start to surface, it's snack time.

This book offers you one hundred deliciously low-carb recipes to choose from, as well as nutritional and allergy-related information, so you can make an informed choice. Need fuel for a road race? At home or on the go? Want to sip your snack? Need a nut-free nosh? This book has you covered.

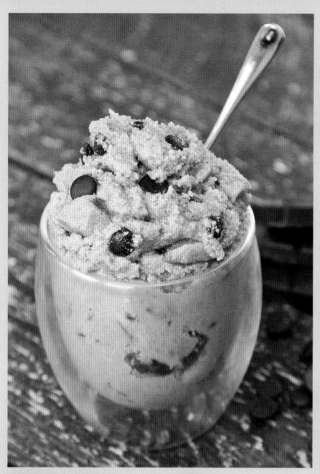

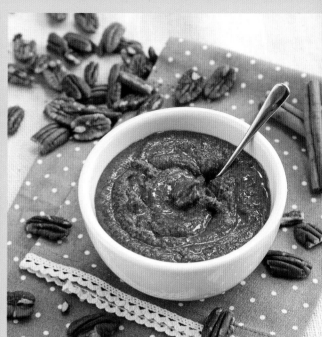

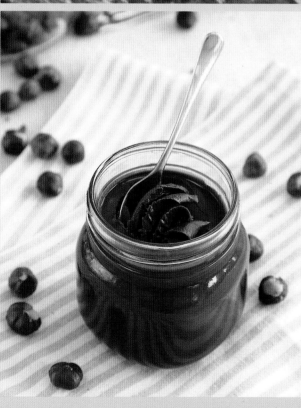

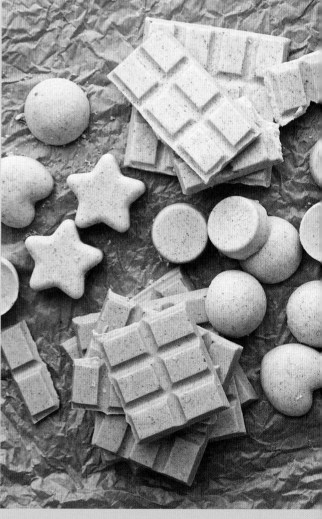

1

THE BASICS:
Versatile, Homemade Nut Butters and Sugar-Free Chocolates

Before you start creating low-carb snacks, including fat bombs, you'll need to make a few simple-to-prepare, basic ingredients, such as nut and seed butters and homemade chocolate. Most nut and seed butters can be kept at room temperature for a few days, and will last for several weeks in a sealed glass jar in the refrigerator. You can also freeze nut and seed butters for 3 to 4 months. Homemade chocolate will keep refrigerated for up to 3 months. The best part is, in addition to being delicious, all these recipes are sugar free.

Almond and Cashew Butter 10

Coconut and Pecan Butter 11

Chocolate-Hazelnut Butter 12

Eggnog-Macadamia Butter 14

White Chocolate and Macadamia Butter 15

Berry Nut Butter 15

Spiced Maple and Pecan Butter 16

Chocolate Chip Cookie Butter 18

Pistachio-Coconut Butter 20

Pumpkin Sun Butter 21

Almond Bliss Butter 22

Homemade Dark Chocolate Three Ways 24

Homemade White Chocolate 27

Almond and Cashew Butter

This delicious spread is a great paleo alternative to peanut butter.

1 cup (150 g /5.3 oz) almonds, blanched or whole

⅓ cup (50 g /1.8 oz) cashews

4 tablespoons (60 ml /2 fl oz) almond oil or macadamia nut oil

Pinch salt (optional)

Seeds from 1 vanilla bean (optional)

½ teaspoon ground cinnamon (optional)

—

Yield: about 1 cup (250 g/8.8 oz)

NUTRITIONAL FACTS
PER SERVING (230G)

Per serving (2 tablespoons [1.1 ounce, or 32 g]): total carbs: 5.5 g; fiber: 2.1 g; net carbs: 3.4 g; protein: 5.2 g; fat: 19.4 g; energy: 205 kcal.

Macronutrient ratio: calories from carbs: 6 percent; protein: 10 percent; fat: 84 percent.

Preheat the oven to 350°F (175°C, or gas mark 4). Spread the almonds and cashews on a baking sheet and place in the preheated oven for 12 to 15 minutes. Watch carefully to prevent burning. Remove from the oven and cool.

In a food processor, pulse the nuts until smooth (or reserve some chopped nuts to add later for a chunkier texture). Depending on your processor, this may take some time. At first, the mixture will be dry. Scrape down the sides several times with a rubber spatula if the mixture sticks.

Add the oil. Continue to blend until you reach the desired consistency. The oil makes the butter smoother and more suitable for creating fat bombs. Add the salt and vanilla bean seeds or cinnamon (if using) and pulse to combine. Spoon the butter into a glass container. Seal and store at room temperature for up to 1 week or refrigerate for up to 3 months.

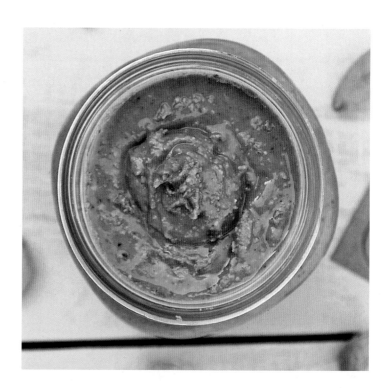

Coconut and Pecan Butter

Keep a napkin handy. You'll drool over this cinnamon-spiced nut butter. Made with pecans and coconut, it's perfect for making chocolate treats.

2 cups (150 g/5.3 oz) unsweetened shredded coconut

1 cup (100 g/3.5 oz) pecans

1 teaspoon sugar-free vanilla extract or ½ teaspoon vanilla powder

1 teaspoon ground cinnamon

¼ teaspoon salt

—
Yield: about 1 cup (250 g/8.8 oz)

In a food processor, combine the coconut, pecans, vanilla, cinnamon, and salt. Pulse until smooth and creamy. Depending on your processor, this may take a few minutes. At first, the mixture will be dry. Scrape down the sides several times with a rubber spatula if the mixture sticks.

Spoon the butter into a glass container. Seal and store at room temperature for up to 1 week or refrigerate for up to 3 months.

NUTRITIONAL FACTS

Per serving (2 tablespoons [1.1 ounce, or 32g]): total carbs: 6.5 g; fiber: 4.4 g; net carbs: 2.1 g; protein: 5 g; fat: 11.6 g; energy: 154 kcal.

Macronutrient ratio: calories from carbs: 6 percent; protein: 15 percent; fat: 79 percent.

To enhance this butter's flavor, use roasted pecans and coconut: Preheat the oven to 350°F (175°C, or gas mark 4). Spread the coconut and pecans on a baking sheet. Place in the preheated oven and roast for 5 to 8 minutes, or until the coconut is lightly golden. Stir once or twice to prevent burning.

Chocolate-Hazelnut Butter

This healthy, low-carb alternative to Nutella is just the thing for making truffles, and it's also great in smoothies.

1 cup (150 g/5.3 oz) hazelnuts

1 cup (130 g/4.6 oz) macadamia nuts

½ cup (75 g/2.6 oz) almonds

1 bar (100 g/3.5 oz) extra-dark chocolate, 85 percent cacao or more

1 tablespoon (15 g/0.5 oz) coconut oil

1 tablespoon (5 g/0.2 oz) unsweetened cacao powder

1 teaspoon sugar-free vanilla extract or ½ teaspoon vanilla powder

2 tablespoons (20 g/0.7 oz) erythritol or Swerve, powdered

Few drops liquid stevia, to taste (optional)

½ cup (120 ml/4 fl oz) coconut milk or heavy whipping cream (optional)

—
Yield: about 2 cups (500 g/1.1 lbs)

Preheat the oven to 375°F (190°C, or gas mark 5). Spread the hazelnuts, macadamia nuts, and almonds on a baking sheet. Place in the preheated oven and bake for about 10 minutes, or until lightly browned. Remove the nuts from the oven and cool for 15 minutes.

Meanwhile, melt the dark chocolate and coconut oil in a double boiler, or heat-proof bowl placed over a small pot filled with 1 cup (235 ml) of boiling water, making sure the water doesn't touch the bottom of the bowl. Stir until melted.

Rub the hazelnuts together in your hands to remove the skins. This makes the butter smooth and avoids the bitter taste imparted by the skins. Place all of the nuts into a food processor and pulse until smooth.

Add the cacao powder, vanilla, erythritol, and stevia (if using) to the melted chocolate. Pour the mixture into the processor with the nuts and pulse until smooth. If you're using the coconut milk, add it to the processor and pulse again.

Transfer the butter to a glass container. Seal and refrigerate for up to 3 months, or 4 weeks if using coconut milk or cream.

NUTRITIONAL FACTS

Per serving (2 tablespoons [1.1 ounce, or 32 g]): total carbs: 5.9 g; fiber: 2.9 g; net carbs: 3 g; protein: 3.9 g; fat: 18.7 g; energy: 193 kcal.

Macronutrient ratio: calories from carbs: 6 percent; protein: 8 percent; fat: 86 percent.

NOTE:

To powder the erythritol, place it in a clean blender or coffee grinder and pulse until powdery, about 15 to 20 seconds.

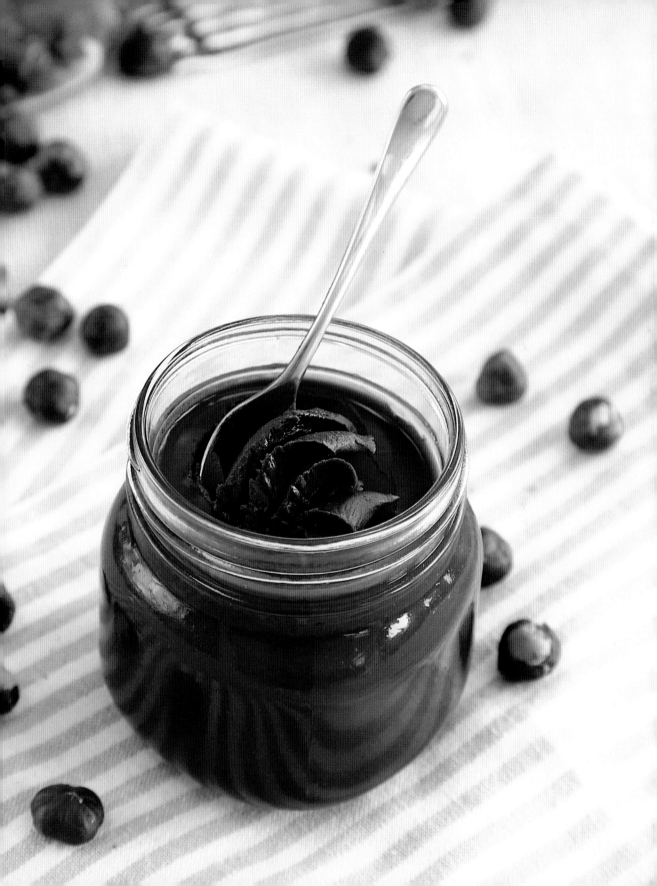

Eggnog-Macadamia Butter

Enjoy the flavors of the holiday season all year 'round! This macadamia-based butter is lightly spiced, creamy, and addictive.

2 cups (260 g/9.2 oz) macadamia nuts

1 teaspoon ground nutmeg

½ teaspoon sugar-free vanilla extract or ¼ teaspoon vanilla powder

½ teaspoon ground cinnamon

½ teaspoon natural rum extract

2 tablespoons (20 g/0.8 oz) erythritol or Swerve, powdered

Few drops liquid stevia, to taste (optional)

—
Yield: about 1¼ cups (290 g/10.2 oz)

In a food processor, combine the macadamia nuts, nutmeg, vanilla, cinnamon, rum extract, and erythritol. Add a few drops of stevia (if using). Process until smooth. The exact amount of time depends on your processor. Spoon the butter into a glass container. Seal and store at room temperature for up to 1 week or refrigerate for up to 3 months.

NUTRITIONAL FACTS

Per serving (2 tablespoons [32 g/ 1.1 oz]): total carbs: 4.6 g; fiber: 2.8 g; net carbs: 1.8 g; protein: 2.3 g; fat: 21.7 g; energy: 209 kcal.

Macronutrient ratio: calories from carbs: 3 percent; protein: 4 percent; fat: 93 percent.

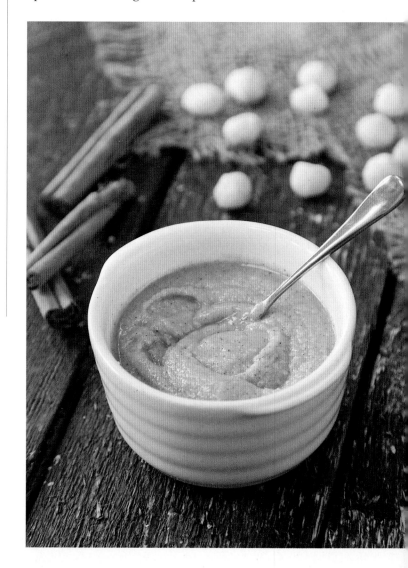

White Chocolate and Macadamia Butter

This recipe combines some of the healthiest high-fat foods in a single jar of goodness: macadamia nuts, coconut butter, and cacao butter. The result? A white chocolate treat that's good for you, too.

1 cup (130 g/4.7 oz) macadamia nuts

½ cup (125 g/4.4 oz) coconut butter

½ cup (110 g/3.9 oz) cacao butter

2 teaspoons sugar-free vanilla extract or 1 teaspoon vanilla powder

¼ cup (40 g/1.4 oz) erythritol or Swerve, powdered

Few drops liquid stevia, to taste (optional)

—

Yield: about 1⅔ cups (410 g/14.5 oz)

In a food processor, combine the macadamia nuts, coconut butter, cacao butter, vanilla, and erythritol. Add the stevia (if using), and process until smooth. The exact amount of time depends on your processor. Spoon the butter into a glass container. Seal and store at room temperature for up to 1 week or refrigerate for up to 3 months.

NUTRITIONAL FACTS

Per serving (2 tablespoons [1.1 ounce, or 32 g]): total carbs: 3.7 g; fiber: 2.4 g; net carbs: 1.3 g; protein: 1.4 g; fat: 21.8 g; energy: 207 kcal.

Macronutrient ratio: calories from carbs: 2 percent; protein: 3 percent; fat: 95 percent.

Berry Nut Butter

Brighten the flavor of your fat bombs with this luscious and fruity Berry Nut Butter.

¾ cup (110 g/3.9 oz) blanched almonds

⅔ cup (90 g/3.2 oz) macadamia nuts

½ cup (125 g/4.4 oz) coconut butter

½ cup (110 g/3.9 oz) coconut oil

¾ cup (60 g/2.1 oz) freeze-dried berry powder (raspberry, strawberry, blackberry, or blueberry) or equivalent weight of whole freeze-dried berries

Few drops liquid stevia, to taste (optional)

—

Yield: about 2 cups (500 g/8.8 oz)

In a food processor, combine the almonds, macadamia nuts, and coconut butter. Add the stevia (if using), and process until smooth. The exact amount of time depends on your processor.

Add the coconut oil and berry powder. Pulse again until combined. Spoon the butter into a glass container. Seal and store for 1 week at room temperature or refrigerate for up to 3 months. Note that the butter will become liquid at room temperature.

NUTRITIONAL FACTS

Per serving (2 tablespoons [1.1 ounce, or 32 g]): total carbs: 6.4 g; fiber: 3.6 g; net carbs: 2.7 g; protein: 2.8 g; fat: 19.7 g; energy: 197 kcal.

Macronutrient ratio: calories from carbs: 5 percent; protein: 6 percent; fat: 89 percent.

Create your own nut butter creations by replacing the berry powder with these alternatives: ¼ cup (25 g/0.9 oz) of beetroot powder, 1 to 2 tablespoons (8 to 16 g/0.3 to 0.6 oz) of pumpkin spice mix, or 1 to 2 teaspoons of turmeric.

Spiced Maple and Pecan Butter

The combination of maple, pecan, and cinnamon smacks of a cool, crisp fall morning, and this sugar-free nut butter captures those rich, spicy flavors to enjoy any time.

3 cups (300 g/10.6 oz) pecans

1 to 2 teaspoons natural maple extract

½ teaspoon ground cinnamon

1 teaspoon sugar-free vanilla extract or ½ teaspoon vanilla powder

Pinch salt

—

Yield: about 1¼ cups (310 g/10.9 oz)

In a food processor, combine the pecans, maple extract, cinnamon, vanilla, and salt. Process until smooth. The exact amount of time depends on your processor. Spoon the butter into a glass container. Seal and store at room temperature for up to 1 week or refrigerate for up to 3 months.

NUTRITIONAL FACTS

Per serving (2 tablespoons [1.1 ounce, or 32g]): total carbs: 4.6 g; fiber: 3.1 g; net carbs: 1.4 g; protein: 2.9 g; fat: 22.3 g; energy: 216 kcal.

Macronutrient ratio: calories from carbs: 3 percent; protein: 5 percent; fat: 92 percent.

NOTE:

For fat bomb-friendly food extracts, use unsweetened food extracts that are free from propylene glycol and any added sugar. Other common ingredients found in food extracts include water, natural oils, alcohol, and glycerin. Avoid using alcohol if your primary aim is to lose weight, but small amounts in food extracts won't do any harm. Another ingredient that turns up is glycerin, which is a liquid byproduct of making soap. It belongs to a special category of carbohydrates called polyols. Glycerin has a minimal effect on blood sugar levels and can be used in small quantities. Certain food extracts can also be swapped for a few drops of essential oils, such as orange, lemon, and mint.

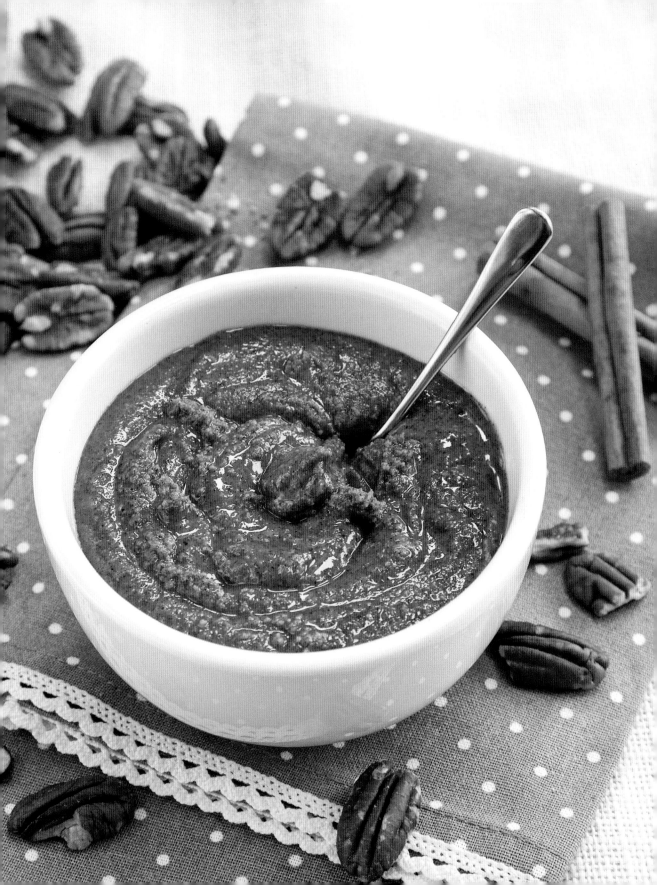

Chocolate Chip Cookie Butter

There's no need to say goodbye to cookies—or chocolate—when you're eating low carb. This decadent butter is the proof, and it's sure to become an absolute favorite!

FOR COOKIES:

1½ cups (150 g/5.3 oz) almond flour

⅓ cup (50 g/1.8 oz) erythritol or Swerve

½ teaspoon baking soda mixed with 1 teaspoon cream of tartar, or 1 teaspoon gluten-free baking powder

Pinch salt

1 teaspoon sugar-free vanilla extract or ½ teaspoon vanilla powder

1 teaspoon freshly grated lemon zest

2 large egg yolks

2 tablespoons (30 g/1.1 oz) butter or ghee, at room temperature

FOR COOKIE BUTTER:

Crushed cookies (recipe follows)

½ cup (112 g/4 oz) unsalted butter or ghee or coconut oil, at room temperature

½ cup (90 g/3.2 oz) dark chocolate chips, 85 percent cacao solids or more, or make your own (see Homemade Dark Chocolate [page 24])

Few drops liquid stevia, to taste (optional)

—
Yield: about 1 cups (470 g/16.6 oz)

Preheat the oven to 300°F (150°C, or gas mark 2).

To make the cookies: In a mixing bowl, combine the almond flour, erythritol, baking soda and cream of tartar, and salt. Mix well to combine. Add the vanilla, lemon zest, egg yolks, and butter. Mix together well with your hands.

Place the dough on a sheet of parchment paper. Top with another sheet of parchment and roll out to create a large cookie about ¼ inch (6.5 mm) thick. Transfer to a baking sheet and it in the preheated oven. Bake for 12 to 15 minutes, or until lightly browned and crispy. Remove from the oven and cool to room temperature. When cool, break into smaller pieces.

To make the cookie butter: In a food processor, pulse together the cookie pieces and butter until smooth. Add the chocolate chips. For a sweeter taste, add the stevia (if using). Pulse quickly to combine. Transfer to a sealed container and refrigerate for up to 1 week.

NOTE:

Instead of vanilla extract and lemon, try cinnamon or pumpkin spice mix and freshly grated orange zest.

NUTRITIONAL FACTS

Per serving (2 tablespoons [1.1 ounce, or 32 g]): total carbs: 3.9 g; fiber: 1.5 g; net carbs: 2.4 g; protein: 3.3 g; fat: 16.6 g; energy: 170 kcal.

Macronutrient ratio: calories from carbs: 6 percent; protein: 8 percent; fat: 87 percent.

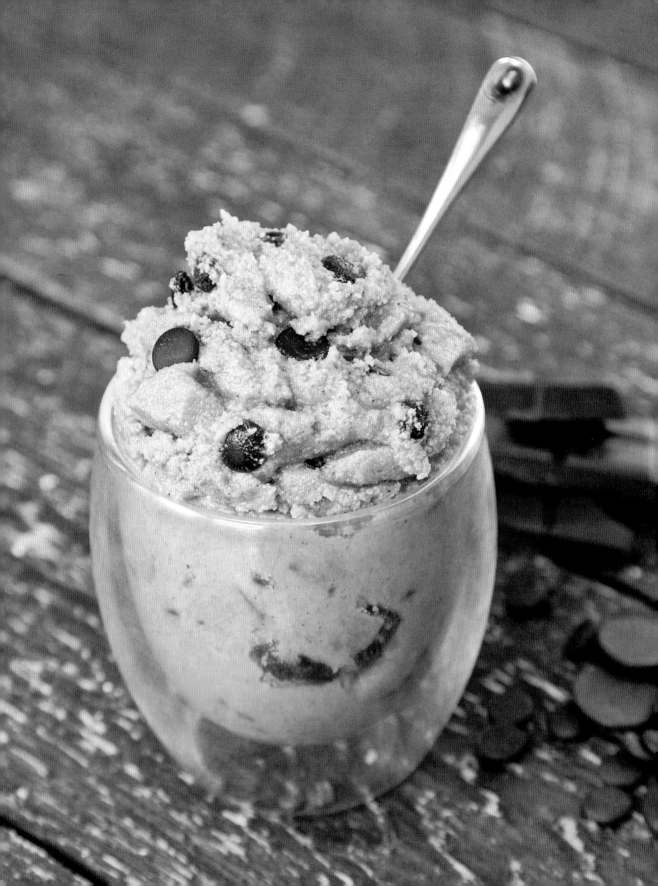

Pistachio-Coconut Butter

Pistachio nuts are like potato chips—it's impossible to eat just one. Get your fix with this creamy nut butter that's packed with pistachios, macadamia nuts, and coconut.

1 cup (120 g/4.2 oz) pistachio nuts

1 cup (75 g/2.6 oz) shredded unsweetened coconut

1 cup (130 g/4.7 oz) macadamia nuts

1 teaspoon sugar-free vanilla extract or ½ teaspoon vanilla powder

Pinch salt

—
Yield: about 1⅓ cups (330 g/11.6 oz)

NUTRITIONAL FACTS

Per serving (2 tablespoons [1.1 ounce, or 32 g]): total carbs: 6.7 g; fiber: 3.5 g; net carbs: 3.2 g; protein: 4.8 g; fat: 15.8 g; energy: 182 kcal.

Macronutrient ratio: calories from carbs: 7 percent; protein: 11 percent; fat: 82 percent.

In a food processor, combine the pistachios, coconut, macadamia nuts, vanilla, and salt. Pulse until smooth. The exact amount of time depends on your processor. Spoon the butter into a glass container. Seal and store at room temperature for up to 1 week or refrigerate for up to 3 months.

NOTE:

Intensify the flavor of this butter by using toasted pistachios, macadamias, and coconut. Preheat the oven to 350°F (175°C, or gas mark 4). Spread the pistachios, macadamias, and coconut on a baking sheet. Place it in the preheated oven and toast for 5 to 8 minutes, or until the coconut is lightly golden. Stir once or twice to prevent burning. The pistachios will turn light brown, instead of green, and the flavor will be more intense.

Pumpkin Sun Butter

Can't eat nuts? Never fear: you can still make fat bombs with this spiced, nut-free seed butter.

1½ cups (210 g/7.4 oz) sunflower seeds

½ cup (65 g/2.3 oz) pumpkin seeds

2 teaspoons ground cinnamon

Pinch salt

—
Yield: about 1¼ cups (280 g/9.9 oz)

In a food processor, combine the sunflower seeds, pumpkin seeds, cinnamon, and salt. Pulse until smooth. The exact amount of time depends on your processor. Spoon the butter into a glass container. Seal and store at room temperature for up to 1 week, or refrigerate for up to 3 months.

NUTRITIONAL FACTS

Per serving (2 tablespoons [1.1 ounce, or 32 g): total carbs: 6.1 g; fiber: 2.8 g; net carbs: 3.3 g; protein: 7.3 g; fat: 16 g; energy: 183 kcal.

Macronutrient ratio: calories from carbs: 7 percent; protein: 16 percent; fat: 77 percent.

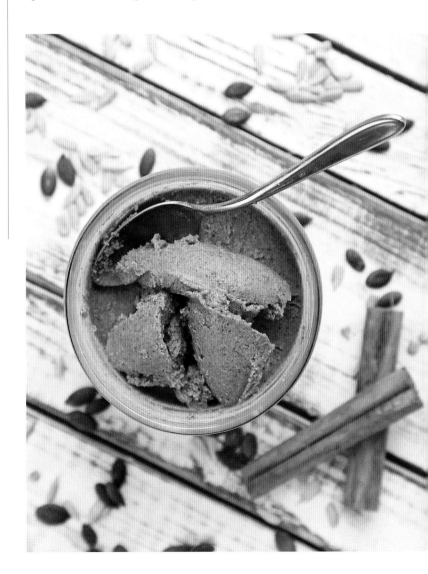

Almond Bliss Butter

This treat will remind you of those fun-size candy bars you got in your Halloween goodie bag. If you adored those chocolate-coated, almond-studded delights, you'll feel like a kid again when you try this rich, delicious nut butter.

2 cups (150 g/5.3 oz) unsweetened shredded coconut

½ cup (75 g/2.6 oz) almonds

2.5 ounces (70 g) dark chocolate, 85 percent cacao solids or more

2.5 ounces (70 g) cacao butter

¼ cup (40 g/1.4 oz) erythritol or Swerve

Few drops liquid stevia, to taste (optional)

—

Yield: about 1⅔ cups (405 g/14.3 oz)

Preheat the oven to 350°F (175°C, or gas mark 4). Spread the coconut and almonds on a baking sheet. Place it in the preheated oven and roast for 5 to 8 minutes, or until the coconut is lightly golden. Stir once or twice to prevent burning. Remove from the oven and set aside for a few minutes to cool.

In a food processor, combine the coconut, almonds, dark chocolate, cacao butter, and erythritol. Pulse until smooth. The exact amount of time depends on your processor. Add the stevia (if using), and pulse again. Spoon the butter into a glass container. Seal and store at room temperature for up to 1 week, or refrigerate for up to 3 months.

NUTRITIONAL FACTS

Per serving (2 tablespoons [1.1 ounce, or 32 g]): total carbs: 5.9 g; fiber: 3.2 g; net carbs: 2.8 g; protein: 4.4 g; fat: 11.8 g; energy: 147 kcal.

Macronutrient ratio: calories from carbs: 8 percent; protein: 12 percent; fat: 80 percent.

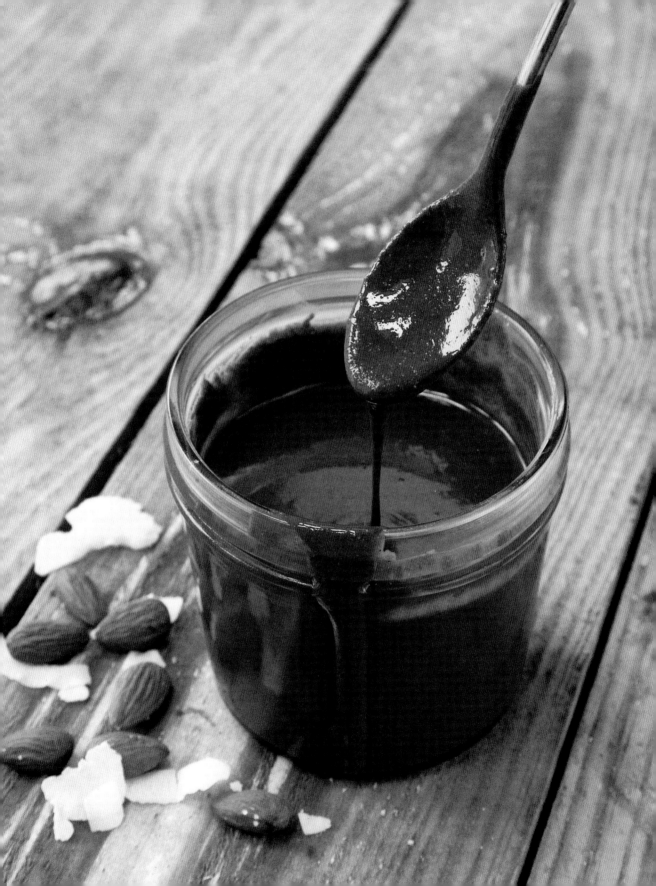

Homemade Dark Chocolate Three Ways

Make healthy, sugar-free chocolate in a few simple steps.

FOR DARK CHOCOLATE USING UNSWEETENED CHOCOLATE (MAKES 8 OUNCES, OR 225 G):

3 ounces (85 g) unsweetened chocolate

3 ounces (85 g) cacao butter

⅓ cup (50 g/1.8 oz) erythritol or Swerve, powdered

1 teaspoon sugar-free vanilla extract or ½ teaspoon vanilla powder

Pinch salt

Few drops liquid stevia, to taste (optional)

—

Yield: dark chocolate using unsweetened chocolate: 8 ounces, or 225

FOR DARK CHOCOLATE USING CACAO POWDER (MAKES 7.5 OUNCES, OR 210 G):

4 ounces (112 g) cacao butter

½ cup (40 g/1.4 oz) unsweetened cacao powder

⅓ cup (50 g/1.8 oz) erythritol or Swerve, powdered

1 teaspoon sugar-free vanilla extract or ½ teaspoon vanilla powder

Pinch salt

Few drops liquid stevia, to taste (optional)

—

Yield: dark chocolate using cacao powder: 7.5 ounces, or 213 g

FOR DARK CHOCOLATE USING COCONUT OIL (MAKES 6.8 OUNCES, OR 195 G):

½ cup (110 g/3.9 oz) coconut oil

½ cup (40 g/1.5 oz) unsweetened cacao powder

¼ cup (40 g/1.4 oz) erythritol or Swerve, powdered

1 teaspoon sugar-free vanilla extract or ½ teaspoon vanilla powder

Pinch salt

Few drops liquid stevia, to taste (optional)

—

Yield: dark chocolate using coconut oil: 6.8 ounces, or 195 g

NUTRITIONAL FACTS

Per serving of each type (1 ounce, or 28 g): total carbs: 3 g/3.5 g/3.7 g; fiber: 1.5 g/1.8 g/1.9 g; net carbs: 1.5 g/1.7 g/1.8 g; protein: 1.5 g/1.1 g/1.1 g; fat: 16.2 g/15.9 g/16.4 g; energy: 164 kcal/150 kcal/151 kcal.

Macronutrient ratio: calories from carbs: 6 percent/5 percent/5 percent; protein: 4 percent/3 percent/3 percent; fat: 92 percent/93 percent/93 percent.

TO MAKE DARK CHOCOLATE USING UNSWEETENED CHOCOLATE: Melt the unsweetened chocolate and cacao butter in a double boiler, or heat-proof bowl placed over a small saucepan filled with 1 cup (235 ml) of water, over medium heat. Remove from the heat and set aside. Stir in the erythritol, vanilla, and salt. If you want a sweeter taste, add the stevia. Pour the chocolate into candy or chocolate molds or onto a parchment-lined baking sheet. Let it harden at room temperature, or in the refrigerator. Remove from the molds. Store at room temperature or refrigerate for up to 3 months.

TO MAKE DARK CHOCOLATE USING CACAO POWDER: Melt the cacao butter in a double boiler, or heat-proof bowl placed over a small saucepan filled with 1 cup (235 ml) of water, over medium heat. Remove from the heat and set aside. Stir in the cacao powder, erythritol, vanilla, and salt. If you want a sweeter taste, add the stevia. Pour into candy or chocolate molds and harden at room temperature or in the refrigerator. Once hardened, remove from the molds and keep in an airtight container. Store at room temperature or refrigerate for up to 3 months.

TO MAKE DARK CHOCOLATE USING COCONUT OIL: Melt the coconut oil in a double boiler, or heat-proof bowl placed over a small saucepan filled with 1 cup (235 ml) of water, over medium heat. Once melted, add the cacao powder, erythritol, vanilla, and salt. If you want a sweeter taste, add the stevia. Pour into candy or chocolate molds and harden in the refrigerator. Once hardened, remove from the molds and store in an airtight container. Always store in the refrigerator: coconut oil melts at room temperature. Refrigerate for up to 3 months or freeze for up to 6 months.

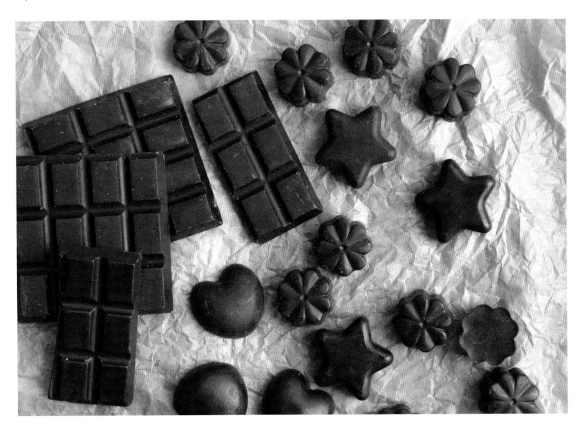

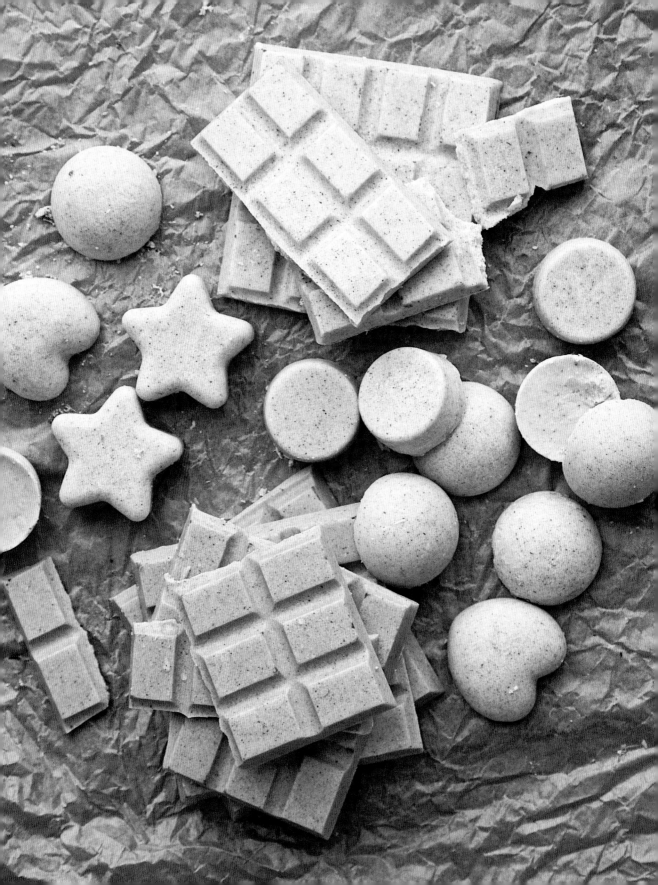

Homemade White Chocolate

Packed with healthy fats and made from real food ingredients (no additives here!), this Homemade White Chocolate is sugar-free and infused with fragrant vanilla.

6 ounces (170 g) cacao butter

1 cup (120 g/4.2 oz) coconut milk powder

⅓ cup (50 g/1.8 oz) erythritol or Swerve, powdered

2 teaspoons sugar-free vanilla extract or 1 teaspoon vanilla powder

Pinch salt

Few drops liquid stevia, to taste (optional)

—
Yield: about 12 ounces, or 340 g

NUTRITIONAL FACTS

Per serving (1 ounce, or 28 g): total carbs: 2.7 g; fiber: 0.1 g; net carbs: 2.6 g; protein: 0.7 g; fat: 19.8 g; energy: 191 kcal.

Macronutrient ratio: calories from carbs: 5 percent; protein: 1 percent; fat: 93 percent.

Melt the cacao butter in a double boiler, or heat-proof bowl placed over a small saucepan filled with 1 cup (235 ml) of water, over medium heat. Remove from the heat and set aside. Add the coconut milk powder, and lucuma powder (if using; see Note), erythritol, vanilla, and salt. If you want a sweeter taste, add the stevia. Pour the mixture into a food processor. Pulse for 30 to 60 seconds, or until smooth. Pour into candy or chocolate molds and let the chocolate harden in the refrigerator. Once solid, remove from the molds. Store at room temperature or refrigerate for up to 3 months.

NOTE:

For an extra nutritional boost, swap ½ cup (60g/0.9 oz) of coconut milk powder with ½ cup (40g/1.4 oz) of lucuma powder: What is lucuma powder? Lucuma, a subtropical fruit, is an anti-inflammatory superfood also known as "Gold of the Incas." It's high in carotene, iron, vitamin B3, and fiber, and has a light orange color. The powder made from this fruit adds natural sweetness to the chocolate, and makes it creamier. Keep in mind that lucuma powder has more than twice as many carbs as coconut milk powder, so stick to the suggested amounts. Using lucuma powder in this recipe will result in 4.3 grams of net carbs per serving.

2

SCHOOL AND WORK SNACKS:
Nourishing Noshes to Fuel Your Day

Study after study has shown that consuming high-carbohydrate, high-glycemic foods spikes insulin, leading to a postmeal crash in both energy and focus. Ever wonder why you want to take a nap about an hour after a slice of pizza?

Fortunately, science is homing in on how our food can help us focus.

You may have heard about the importance of protein in our diet, but only recently have we come to understand what a huge role high-protein foods play in our mental health. Studies show that protein improves concentration levels. It elevates dopamine, which regulates happiness, and neurotransmitters that help brain cells "talk" with each other and function properly. Research also suggests that high-protein diets may reduce symptoms of ADHD and improve behavior and attention.

By consuming snacks that include beneficial fatty acids such as omega-3s, which are crucial to a well-functioning brain, concentration can be improved. Because the body can't produce omega 3-s, we need to get them from our diet—walnuts and flaxseeds are great options. One particular type of omega-3 is DHA, which has been shown in some studies to have a direct impact on ADHD and concentration levels.

Likewise, it is hard to stay focused at work or school if your tummy is rumbling. Snacks with a healthy amount of fiber can help you stay satiated for extended periods. Fiber comes in two forms: soluble and insoluble. While insoluble fiber passes through the digestive system relatively untouched, soluble fiber, the kind found in nuts, flaxseeds, and psyllium husk, absorbs water in your stomach and gut, thereby helping you feel full longer.

This chapter contains recipes that are optimized for heightened concentration, a consistent level of energy, and staving off hunger to help you be the best you (and your children, if you have them) can be at work or school. Not just superhealthy, most of these snacks are also nut-free, which make them nice options in "peanut/nut-free" schools or workplaces.

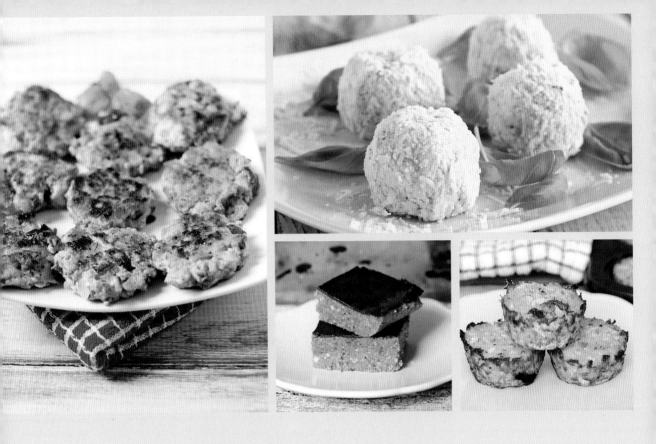

Savory Baked Chicken Nuggets 30

Sun-Dried Tomato Chicken Sliders 32

Italian Meatballs 35

Cauliflower Pizza Bites 36

Herbed Cheese Fat Bombs 38

Salmon Pâté Fat Bombs 40

Chorizo and Avocado Fat Bombs 42

Bacon & Egg Maple Muffins 44

Pumpkin Chocolate Chip Muffins 46

Supersmart Bars 49

Savory Baked Chicken Nuggets

Chicken nuggets are always a favorite with the kids, but you know you love them too! They are supertasty and an excellent source of protein, which keeps that concentration level up all day. Try making a double batch and store them in the freezer in an airtight bag or container.

1 pound (455 g) chicken breasts (about 3 large breasts), cut into bite-size pieces

¼ cup (55 g) grass-fed butter, melted

1 cup (100 g) almond meal or cashew flour

3 tablespoons (24 g) sesame seeds

1 tablespoon (7 g) paprika

2 teaspoons onion powder

1½ teaspoons salt

1 teaspoon garlic powder

¼ teaspoon cayenne pepper

—

Yield: about 24 nuggets

Preheat the oven to 400°F (200°C, or gas mark 6). Place a wire rack in a baking sheet or baking dish. (If you don't have a wire rack, line the baking sheet with parchment paper.)

Place the melted butter in a small bowl. In a separate small bowl, mix together the almond meal, sesame seeds, paprika, onion powder, salt, garlic powder, and cayenne pepper.

Put five or so pieces of chicken in the bowl with butter and coat them well. Then put the chicken into the bowl with the spices and coat evenly. Set the chicken on the wire rack or parchment paper and repeat the process until all of your chicken is coated.

Bake for 10 minutes. Then turn the oven to broil, and bake another 4 or 5 minutes, until golden brown. You don't have to flip them (thanks goodness, because it's a pain!).

Nuggets store well in the fridge for 3 to 4 days or in the freezer for up to 6 months.

NUTRITIONAL FACTS

Per nugget: total carbs: 1.6 g; fiber: 0.8 g; net carbs: 0.8 g; protein: 5.6 g; fat: 5.5 g; calories: 76.

Macronutrient ratio: calories from carbs: 8 percent; protein: 29 percent; fat: 63 percent.

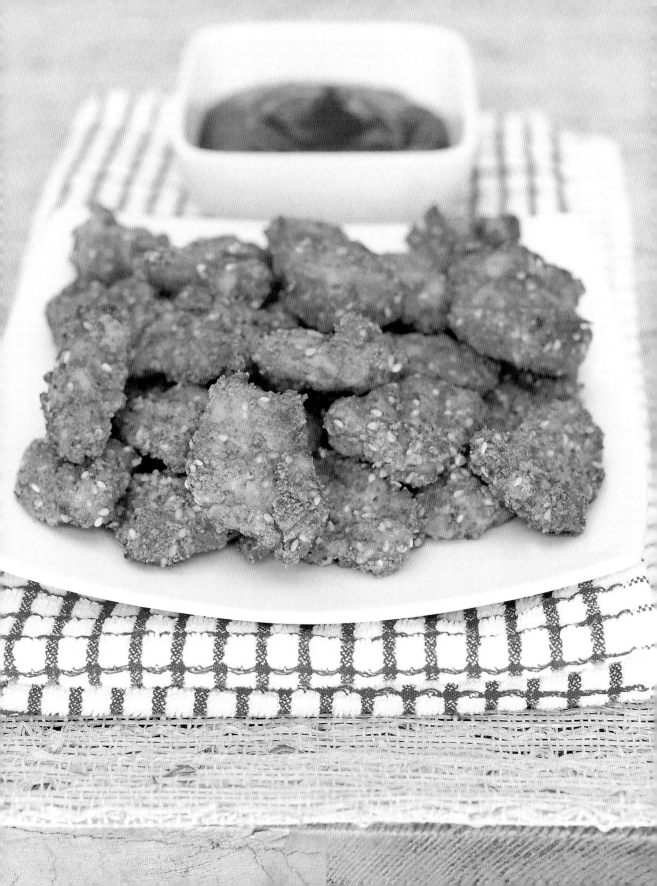

Sun-Dried Tomato Chicken Sliders

This flavorful slider is a fun alternative to a traditional chicken burger. And because it's all protein, it's a great snack to keep your concentration going strong.

1 pound (455 g) ground chicken

½ of a small onion, finely chopped

2 tablespoons (14 g) sundried tomatoes packed in oil, chopped

2 tablespoons (5 g) fresh basil, chopped

2 cloves of garlic, pressed

2 teaspoons salt

1 teaspoon ground black pepper

2 tablespoons (27 g) coconut oil

—
Yield: about 15 sliders

In a medium bowl, combine the chicken, onion, sundried tomatoes, basil, garlic, salt, and pepper until well combined. To form sliders, take a spoonful of the mixture and pat together a patty that is 2 to 3 inches (5 to 7.5 cm) in diameter.

Heat a large pan over medium-high and add the coconut oil. Carefully place patties in the pan, as many as you can without touching. Once the patties start to brown, carefully turn them, and cook for a few more minutes so they can brown. Then turn the heat down to low and cook for about 7 more minutes, or until no longer pink in the middle. Snack on them as is, or turn them into a meal by using them to top a salad.

NUTRITIONAL FACTS

Per slider: total carbs: 0.7 g; fiber: 0.1 g; net carbs: 0.5 g; protein: 5 g; fat: 4 g; calories: 63.

Macronutrient ratio: calories from carbs: 4 percent; protein: 34 percent; fat: 62 percent.

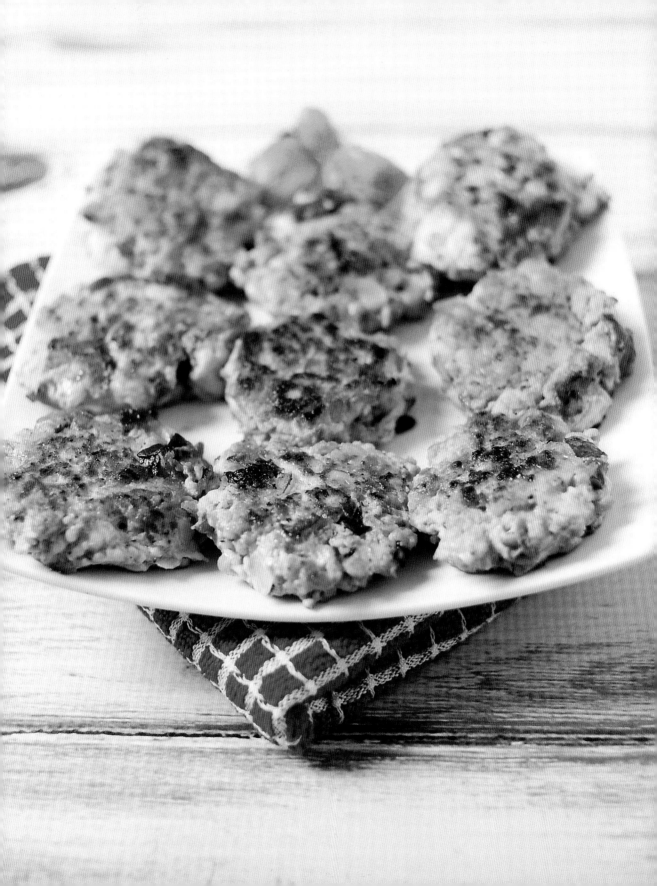

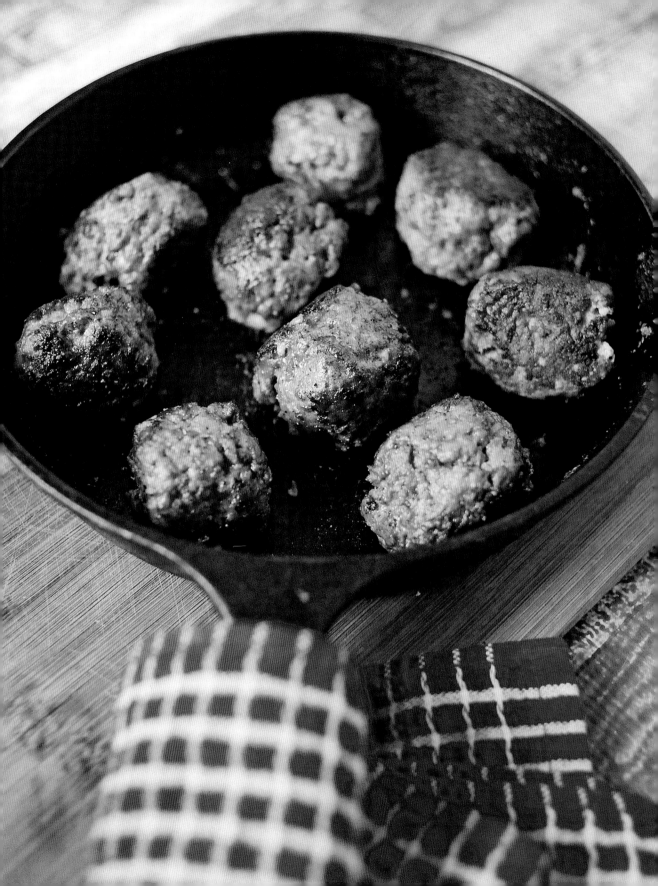

Italian Meatballs

Not only does grass-fed meat contain lots of iron, but it also has many powerful nutrients that help build strong bones and a strong immune system. It also provides a good source of steady energy and concentration, and on top of that, it burns belly fat from its abundant CLA (conjugated linoleic acid), a fatty acid. Talk about a perfect snack. These absolutely delicious meatballs don't need any messy tomato sauce, which makes them perfect for packing.

1 pound (455 g) grass-fed ground beef

½ pound (225 g) ground Italian sausage (removed from casing if needed)

½ of a small onion, finely chopped or grated

2 eggs

2 cloves of garlic, minced

¼ cup (28 g) almond meal or flour

3 tablespoons (12 g) fresh parsley, finely chopped

1 ½ teaspoons salt

1 teaspoon ground black pepper

1 teaspoon dried basil

1 teaspoon dried oregano

—
Yield: about 15 meatballs

Preheat the oven to 350°F (180°C, or gas mark 4).

In a medium bowl, mix together the beef, sausage, onion, eggs, garlic, almond meal, parsley, salt, pepper, basil, and oregano by hand. Form the meatballs about 3 inches (7.5 cm) in diameter.

Add the meatballs to a large cast iron skillet (or other ovenproof skillet) over medium-high heat. Cook until they are browned on all sides. Then place the skillet in the oven (or transfer the meatballs to a baking sheet) and bake for an additional 10 minutes.

NUTRITIONAL FACTS

Per meatball: total carbs: 1.6 g; fiber: 0.4 g; net carbs: 1.3 g; protein: 10.1 g; fat: 9.6 g; calories: 134.

Macronutrient ratio: calories from carbs: 5 percent; protein: 30 percent; fat: 65 percent.

Cauliflower Pizza Bites

This gluten-free pizza crust can be turned into mini, easy-to-eat pizzas. It just so happens that this is the healthiest pizza crust around. With six different types of B vitamins for energy, lots of vitamin C, and a load of antioxidants, this is a super snack.

1 large head of cauliflower, cored and broken into large florets

1 egg

4 ounces (115 g) soft goat cheese (Chevre)

1 tablespoon (3 g) dried oregano

1 teaspoon salt

Optional toppings:

Tomato or pizza sauce

Parmesan or mozzarella cheese

Olives, pepperoni, etc.

—

Yield: 12 pizza bites

NUTRITIONAL FACTS

Per bite: total carbs: 3.7 g; fiber: 1.5 g; net carbs: 2.2 g; protein: 3.6 g; fat: 2.7 g; calories: 50.

Macronutrient ratio: calories from carbs: 28 percent; protein: 27 percent; fat: 45 percent.

Preheat the oven to 400°F (200°C, or gas mark 6). Grease a 12-cup mini-muffin pan.

In a food processor, chop the cauliflower until it is a rice-like consistency. Bring a pot of water to a boil. Add the cauliflower and cook it for 6 to 8 minutes, until soft. Strain and rinse with cold water. Lay out a clean kitchen towel. Pour the "rice" onto the towel, wrap the towel around the "rice," and twist it and squeeze out as much water as you can.

In a medium bowl, beat the egg and add the goat cheese, oregano, and salt. Add the cauliflower "rice" and blend it all together with your hands. It's messy, but it works best this way.

Evenly spoon mixture into the muffin cups, filling them close to the top. Press down the dough evenly and firmly to ensure it sticks together. Bake for 15 to 18 minutes, or until the tops start to turn a light brown. Remove from the oven and let cool in the pan for at least 10 minutes.

Dip in tomato sauce or add whatever toppings you desire.

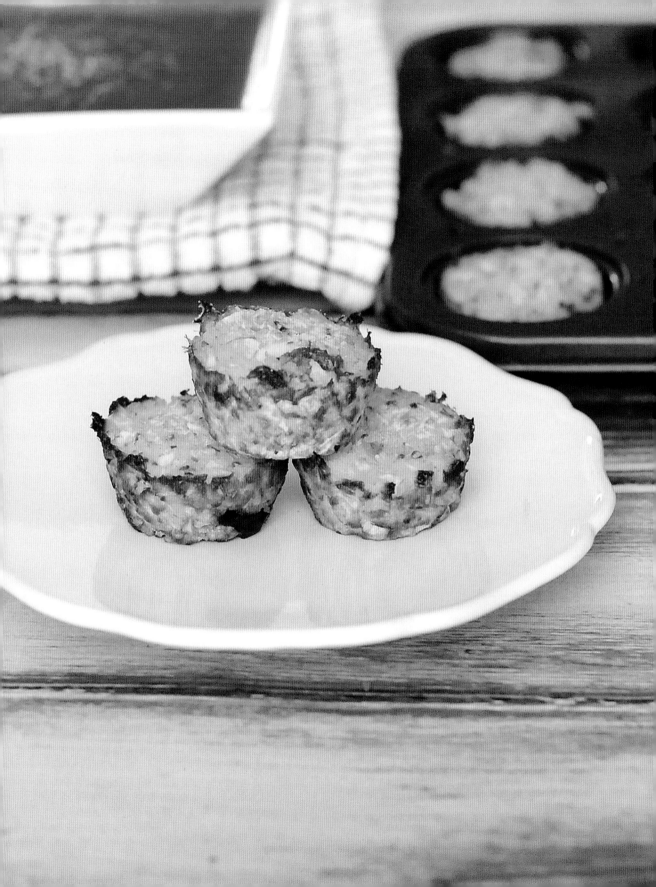

Herbed Cheese Fat Bombs

Reach for one of these cheesy fat bombs the next time you're craving a snack. They're infused with garlic and fresh herbs and coated in Parmesan cheese, and they're incredibly satisfying.

3.5 ounces (100 g) full-fat cream cheese, at room temperature

¼ cup (56 g/2 oz) unsalted butter, at room temperature

4 pieces (12 g /0.4 oz) sun-dried tomatoes, drained and chopped

4 (12 g/0.4 oz) pitted olives, such as kalamatas, chopped

2 to 3 tablespoons (10 g/0.4 oz) chopped fresh herbs (such as basil, thyme, and oregano), or 2 teaspoons dried herbs

2 cloves of garlic, crushed

Salt and pepper, to taste

5 tablespoons (25 g /0.9 oz) grated Parmesan cheese

—
Yield: 5 servings

In a bowl, mash together the cream cheese and butter, or process in a food processor until smooth.

Add the sun-dried tomatoes, olives, herbs, and garlic. Season with salt and pepper. Mix well to combine. Refrigerate for 20 to 30 minutes, or until set.

Using a large spoon or an ice cream scoop, divide the mixture into five balls. Roll each ball in the Parmesan cheese. Enjoy immediately or refrigerate in an airtight container for up to 1 week.

NUTRITIONAL FACTS

Per serving: total carbs: 2 g; fiber: 0.3 g; net carbs: 1.7 g; protein: 3.7 g; fat: 17.1 g; energy: 164 kcal.

Macronutrient ratio: calories from carbs: 4 percent; protein: 8 percent; fat: 88 percent.

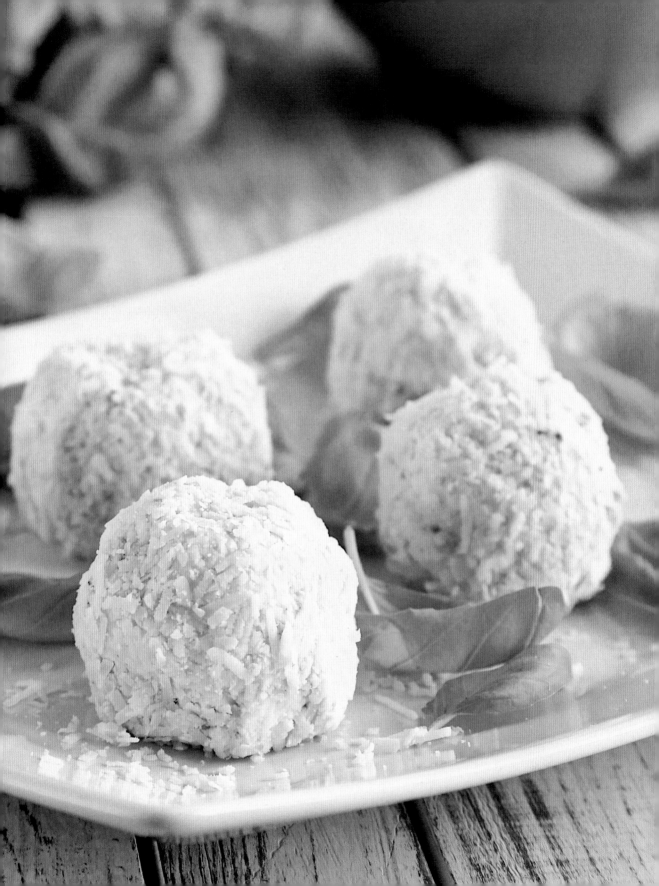

Salmon Pâté Fat Bombs

Smoked salmon and cream cheese—partners in crime—are at their best when dressed up with lemon and dill. This simple recipe shows you how to transform that classic combination into fabulous, keto-friendly fat bombs.

3.5 ounces (100 g) full-fat cream cheese, at room temperature

⅓ cup (75 g /2.7 oz) unsalted butter or ghee, at room temperature

1 small package (50 g /1.8 oz) smoked salmon

1 tablespoon (15 ml/0.5 fl oz) fresh lemon juice

2 tablespoons (8 g/0.3 oz) chopped fresh dill, plus additional for garnishing

Salt and pepper, to taste

Crispy lettuce leaves, for serving (optional)

—
Yield: 6 servings

In a food processor, combine the cream cheese, butter, smoked salmon, lemon juice, and dill. Pulse until smooth.

Line a baking sheet with parchment paper. Spoon about 2 tablespoons (40 g/1.4 oz) of the mixture per portion onto the prepared sheet. Garnish each with more dill. Refrigerate for 20 to 30 minutes, or until set. Alternatively, transfer the mixture to an airtight container and refrigerate. When ready to serve, spoon out 2 tablespoons (40 g/1.4 oz) Per serving and serve on top of lettuce leaves. Keep refrigerated in an airtight container for up to 1 week.

NUTRITIONAL FACTS

Per serving: total carbs: 0.8 g; fiber: 0.1 g; net carbs: 0.7 g; protein: 3.2 g; fat: 15.7 g; energy: 147 kcal

Macronutrient ratio: calories from carbs: 2 percent; protein: 8 percent; fat: 90 percent.

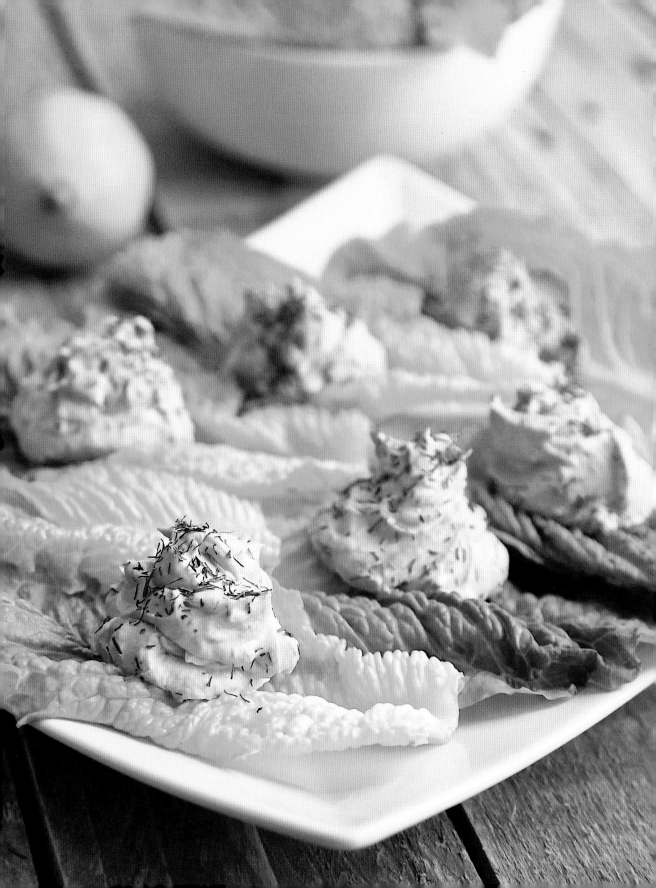

Chorizo and Avocado Fat Bombs

Load crispy bits of chorizo and diced hardboiled eggs into avocado halves for filling fat bombs that double as a quick low-carb lunch or brunch.

3.5 ounces (100 g) Spanish chorizo sausage, diced

2 large hardboiled eggs, cooled, peeled, and diced

¼ cup (56 g /2 oz) unsalted butter, at room temperature

2 tablespoons (30 g/1.1 oz) mayonnaise, preferably homemade

1 tablespoon (15 ml/0.5 fl oz) freshly squeezed lemon juice

2 tablespoons (8 g/0.3 oz) chopped fresh chives

Salt and cayenne pepper, to taste

4 large (400 g /14.1 oz) avocado halves, pitted

—
Yield: 4 servings

In a hot pan, fry the chorizo for a few minutes until crispy. Remove from the heat and set aside.

In a mixing bowl, combine the eggs, chorizo (reserving a small amount for topping), and the butter. Mash together with a fork. Add the mayonnaise, lemon juice, and chives. Season with salt and cayenne pepper. Mix with a fork to combine. Refrigerate for 20 to 30 minutes, or until set.

Just before serving, top each avocado half with one-quarter of the egg and chorizo mixture. Sprinkle with the reserved chorizo and enjoy immediately. Keep the egg and chorizo mixture refrigerated in an airtight container for up to 5 days.

NUTRITIONAL FACTS

Per serving (1 stuffed avocado half): total carbs: 9.5 g; fiber: 6.8 g; net carbs: 2.7 g; protein: 11.4 g; fat: 38.9 g; energy: 419 kcal.

Macronutrient ratio: calories from carbs: 3 percent; protein: 11 percent; fat: 86 percent.

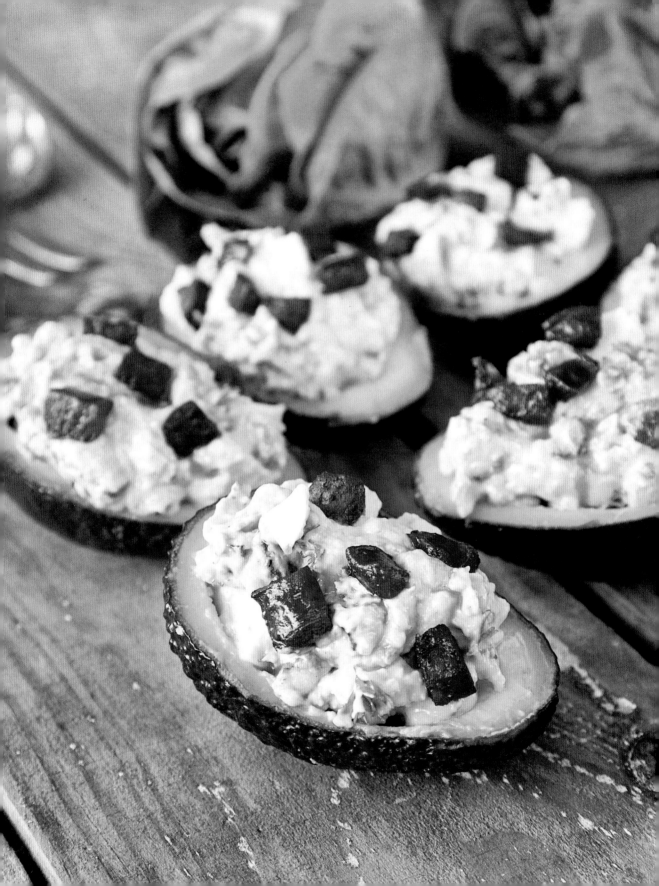

Bacon & Egg Maple Muffins

With a sweet hint of maple and some salty bacon, this delectable snack is superfilling and satisfying. As it's made with an abundance of eggs, considered "brain food" by David Perlmutter, M.D., in his bestselling book *Grain Brain*, this muffin clearly is an ideal snack.

8 to 10 slices nitrate-free bacon

7 eggs, room temperature

¼ cup (55 g) grass-fed butter, melted

2 tablespoons (40 g) maple syrup

½ cup (56 g) coconut flour

½ teaspoon salt

¼ teaspoon baking soda

¼ cup (60 ml) unsweetened canned coconut milk (stirred first)

—

Yield: 12 muffins

NUTRITIONAL FACTS

Per muffin: total carbs: 5.2 g; fiber: 1.7 g; net carbs: 3.5 g; protein: 6.4 g; fat: 10 g; calories: 139.

Macronutrient ratio: calories from carbs: 15 percent; protein: 19 percent; fat: 66 percent.

Preheat the oven to 400°F (200°C, or gas mark 6). Place the bacon on a foil-lined baking sheet and bake for 8 to 10 minutes on each side. You want it to get really brown and crispy!

While the bacon bakes, in a medium bowl, mix together the eggs, butter, coconut milk, and maple syrup. In a small bowl, mix together the coconut flour, salt, and baking soda. Add to the egg mixture and stir well. Make sure you get all of the clumps out from the coconut flour.

When the bacon is done, place it on a paper towel to cool off a bit and then crumble it into the batter.

Reduce the heat to 350°F (180°C, or gas mark 4). Line a 12-cup muffin pan with silicone or paper muffin liners, or grease the cups. Fill the cups about two-thirds full. Bake for 20 minutes, or until a toothpick inserted in the middle of a muffin comes out clean.

These freeze well. Just pull one out the night before and place it in the fridge so it will be ready to go to school/work the next day. They're best when reheated but also yummy when eaten cool or at room temperature.

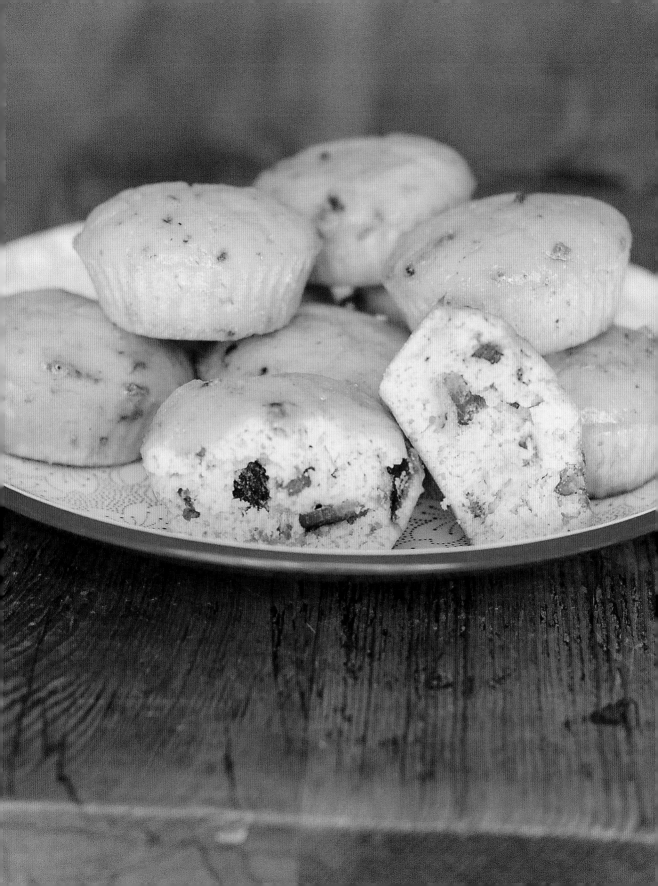

Pumpkin Chocolate Chip Muffins

This fall snack tastes amazing, but is also superhealthy. These muffins have lots of fiber from the coconut flour and pumpkin purée, tons of protein from the eggs, antioxidants from the dark chocolate, and good healthy brain fat from the coconut oil to boot.

¾ cup (84 g) coconut flour

¾ cup (144 g) coconut palm sugar

1 tablespoon (6.6 g) pumpkin pie spice

1 teaspoon ground cinnamon

¾ teaspoon baking soda

½ teaspoon salt

9 eggs, room temperature

⅓ cup (82 g) pumpkin purée

2 tablespoons (40 g) maple syrup

1 teaspoon vanilla extract

2 tablespoons (28 ml) unsweetened canned coconut milk (stirred first)

⅓ cup (80 ml) coconut oil, melted

1 cup (175 g) dark chocolate chips

—
Yield: 18 muffins

Preheat the oven to 350°F (180°C, or gas mark 4). Line eighteen cups of a muffin pan with silicone or paper muffin liners, or grease the cups.

In a medium bowl, mix together the coconut flour, coconut palm sugar, pumpkin pie spice, cinnamon, baking soda, and salt. In another bowl, whisk together the eggs, pumpkin purée, maple syrup, vanilla, and coconut milk. Add the wet ingredients to the dry and mix until well combined. Add the coconut oil and stir until smooth. Fold in the chocolate chips.

Pour the batter into the prepared muffin cups about two-thirds full. Bake for 23 to 25 minutes, or until a toothpick inserted in the middle of a muffin comes out clean, and eat while the chocolate is still melting!

These freeze well for up to 6 months.

NUTRITIONAL FACTS

Per muffin: total carbs: 21.2 g; fiber: 2.1 g; net carbs: 18.2 g; protein: 4.8 g; fat: 11.1 g; calories: 194.

Macronutrient ratio: calories from carbs: 42 percent; protein: 9 percent; fat: 49 percent.

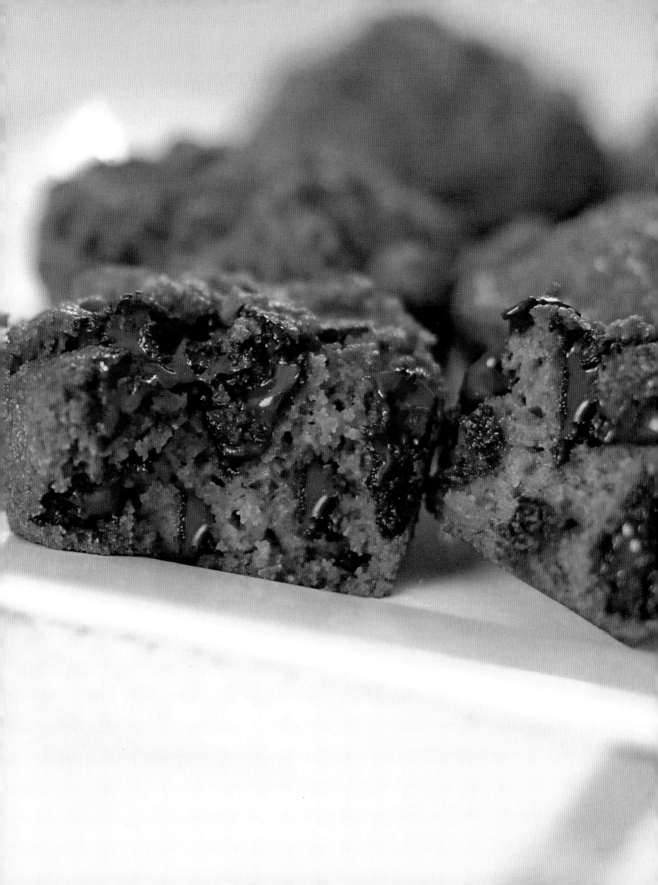

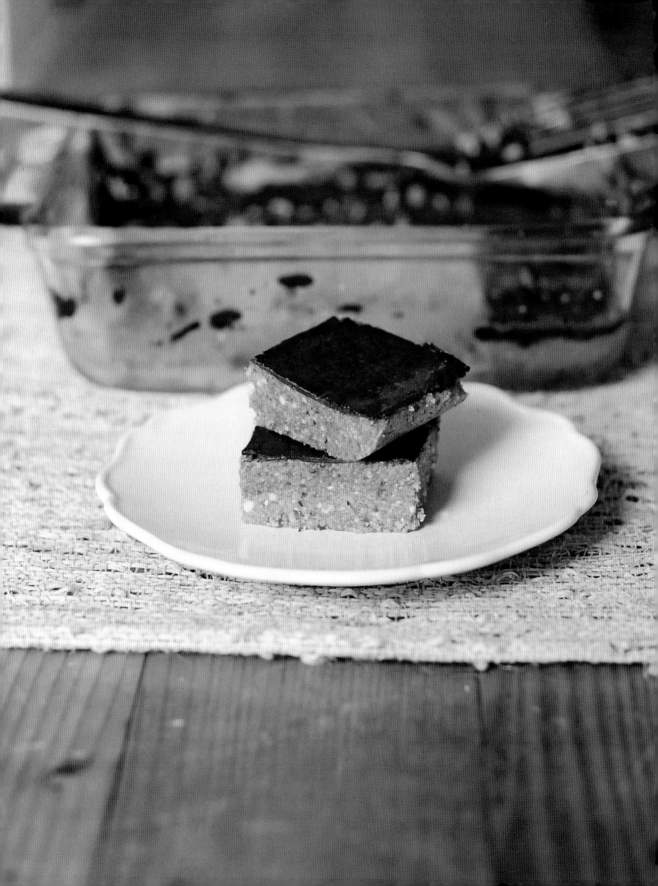

Supersmart Bars

These taste like candy bars! But with the omega-3–rich walnuts, which can help with concentration, and the magnesium-packed cashews, which can help improve memory, this is the exact opposite of a candy bar. Further, the low-glycemic coconut nectar can help stabilize blood sugar levels, while the dark chocolate offers a little mental boost. This is an ideal snack for school or work!

1 cup (120 g) walnuts

1 cup (110 g) cashews

1 cup (80 g) unsweetened shredded coconut

⅔ cup (175 g) almond butter

⅓ cup (144 g) coconut oil

⅓ cup (115 g) coconut nectar

1 tablespoon (15 ml) vanilla extract

½ teaspoon salt

⅓ cup (58 g) dark chocolate chips

—
Yield: 12 bars

In a food processor, blend the walnuts, cashews, coconut, almond butter, coconut oil, coconut nectar, vanilla, and salt until the mixture starts to solidify. Then place the mixture into an 8 x 8 inch (20 x 20 cm) baking dish or pan and press firmly until flat and even. Place in the fridge for 30 to 60 minutes.

Set a small mixing bowl over a small pot of simmering water (be careful that the bowl does not touch the water). Put the chocolate chips in the bowl and stir until melted. Spread the chocolate over the bars and put back in the fridge until it hardens. Cut into 2 x 2 inch (5 x 5 cm) squares. You may want to use a metal spatula to get the squares out. The first one may be tricky to get out but the rest are easy. Store in the fridge.

NUTRITIONAL FACTS

Per bar: total carbs: 14.2 g; fiber: 3.3 g; net carbs: 10.4 g; protein: 6.9 g; fat: 31.2 g; calories: 344.

Macronutrient ratio: calories from carbs: 16 percent; protein: 8 percent; fat: 76 percent.

3

AT-HOME SNACKS:
Skip the Chips for Delicious, Healthy Options

It is four in the afternoon. Dinner isn't for another couple of hours. You and your kids—if you have them—are hungry. You step to the pantry and stare into an unsatisfying abyss of prepackaged saltiness.

Like many people, you tear open a bag of chips or throw popcorn at the problem. The moment that bag rips open, you've lost. The endorphin rush of the first bite will lead to the second, then the third, and before you know it, there is no room left for a healthy dinner.

If any of this sounds familiar, this chapter will change your world.

There is a much healthier, tastier, and more satisfying approach to at-home snacks, and the recipes in this chapter are aimed at turning this traditionally nutritional void into something much more beneficial. All that is needed is less than 10 minutes of prep time and, potentially, a little marketing skill and resolve.

Preparation: If you are making and serving snacks at home, you have the advantage of an oven. Use that advantage to serve aromatic, warm snacks, which are more appetizing than something pulled from a box or bag. Conversely, on a warm summer day, retrieving a cool treat from the fridge will get everyone excited about snack time.

Marketing: Say this aloud: "It isn't a snack, it's an appetizer." After all, who doesn't love appetizers? That's what people eat at restaurants. Appetizers at home? What a delight. Likely, you and/or family will eat more kale chips (or whatever veggie) than if you had set them on their plates at dinnertime. This one is a win-win.

Resolve: Whether it is your family or yourself, change can be a struggle. If the norm is chips, and you prepare something new, don't relent. Let the new snack be the only snack.

A more likely test of your resolve will concern whether these healthy snacks, which are being aggressively devoured, are going to ruin everyone's appetite for dinner. With the veggie "appetizers," you don't have to worry about getting overly stuffed. Unlike traditional processed snacks, whole-food "appetizers" appropriately trigger satiation receptors in the brain so no one will overeat. Worst case, if they do, they will have filled up on nutritious vegetables. That is also a win-win.

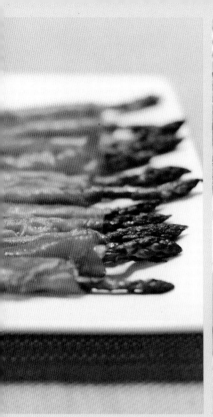
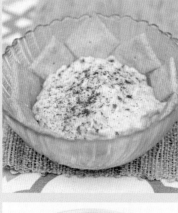
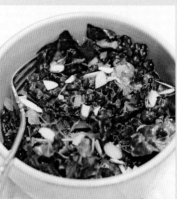
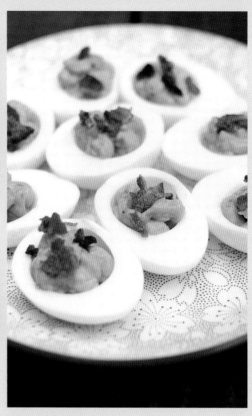

Waldorf Salad Fat Bombs 53

Kale Salad 54

Zesty Walnut Brussels Sprouts 57

Green Deviled Eggs & Bacon 58

Prosciutto-Wrapped Asparagus 60

Cauliflower Hummus 61

Roasted Red Pepper Dip 62

Flatbread "PB&J" 63

Pork Belly Fat Bombs 64

N'Oatmeal Cookies 66

Vanilla-Keto Ice Cream 69

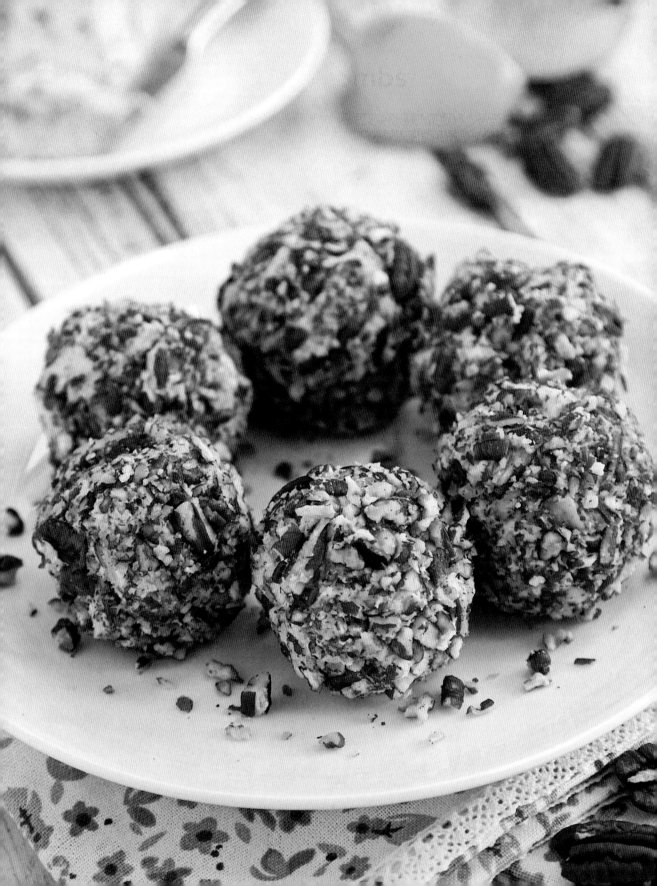

Waldorf Salad Fat Bombs

There's only one thing to do when you've got pecans, cheese, and green apples lurking in your kitchen. Make these sugar-free, bite-size fat bombs!

3 ounces (85 g) full-fat cream cheese, at room temperature

2 tablespoons (28 g/1 oz) unsalted butter or ghee, at room temperature

½ cup (65 g/2.3 oz) crumbled blue cheese

½ of a small (60 g/2.1 oz) green apple, diced into ½ inch (1.5 cm) pieces

¼ teaspoon garlic powder

¼ teaspoon onion powder

2 tablespoons (5 g/0.2 oz) chopped fresh chives or spring onion

Salt and pepper, to taste

⅔ cup (70 g/2.5 oz) pecans or walnuts, roughly chopped

Yield: 6 servings

In a bowl, mash together the cream cheese and butter, or process in a food processor until smooth.

Add the crumbled blue cheese, apple, garlic powder, onion powder, and chives. Stir to combine. Season with salt and pepper. Refrigerate for 20 to 30 minutes, or until set.

Using a large spoon or an ice cream scoop, divide the mixture into six balls. Roll each ball in the pecans. Enjoy immediately or refrigerate in an airtight container for up to 1 week.

NUTRITIONAL FACTS

Per serving: total carbs: 4 g; fiber: 1.5 g; net carbs: 2.5 g; protein: 4.5 g; fat: 19.3 g; energy: 193 kcal.

Macronutrient ratio: calories from carbs: 5 percent; protein: 9 percent; fat: 86 percent.

Kale Salad

Who knew kale could make such a delightfully mild and tasty salad? Because kale leaves don't get soggy and soak in flavor over time, this is a great recipe to make and store in your fridge for a delicious superfood snack any time. To make this salad nut-free, either omit the almonds or substitute roasted pepitas.

FOR SALAD:

1 bunch of Tuscan kale

1½ cups (132 g) brussels sprouts, grated or finely sliced (optional)

3 tablespoons (21 g) sliced almonds

3 tablespoons (23 g) dried cranberries

½ cup (50 g) grated Parmesan cheese

FOR DRESSING:

½ cup (120 ml) extra-virgin olive oil

3 tablespoons (45 ml) fresh lemon juice

1½ tablespoons (23 g) Dijon mustard

1 shallot, minced

2 small cloves of garlic, minced

1 teaspoon salt

Freshly ground black pepper, to taste

—

Yield: 4 servings

TO MAKE THE SALAD: Remove the stems from the kale and roughly chop the leaves. You should have about 4 cups (220 g). Place in a large mixing bowl. Add the brussels sprouts, if using, along with the almonds, cranberries, and Parmesan.

TO MAKE THE DRESSING: In a small bowl, mix together the olive oil, lemon juice, mustard, shallot, garlic, salt, and pepper. Pour the dressing over the kale mixture, and toss well. Let marinate in the fridge for at least 1 hour.

The salad lasts, covered, about 3 days in the fridge.

NUTRITIONAL FACTS

Per serving (w/o brussels sprouts): total carbs: 10.1 g; fiber: 1.3 g; net carbs: 8.5 g; protein: 4.7 g; fat: 33.2 g; calories: 345.

Macronutrient ratio: calories from carbs: 11 percent; protein: 5 percent; fat: 83 percent.

Per serving (w/ brussels sprouts): total carbs: 13.1 g; fiber: 2.6 g; net carbs: 10.2 g; protein: 5.8 g; fat: 33.3 g; calories: 359.

Macronutrient ratio: calories from carbs: 14 percent; protein: 6 percent; fat: 80 percent.

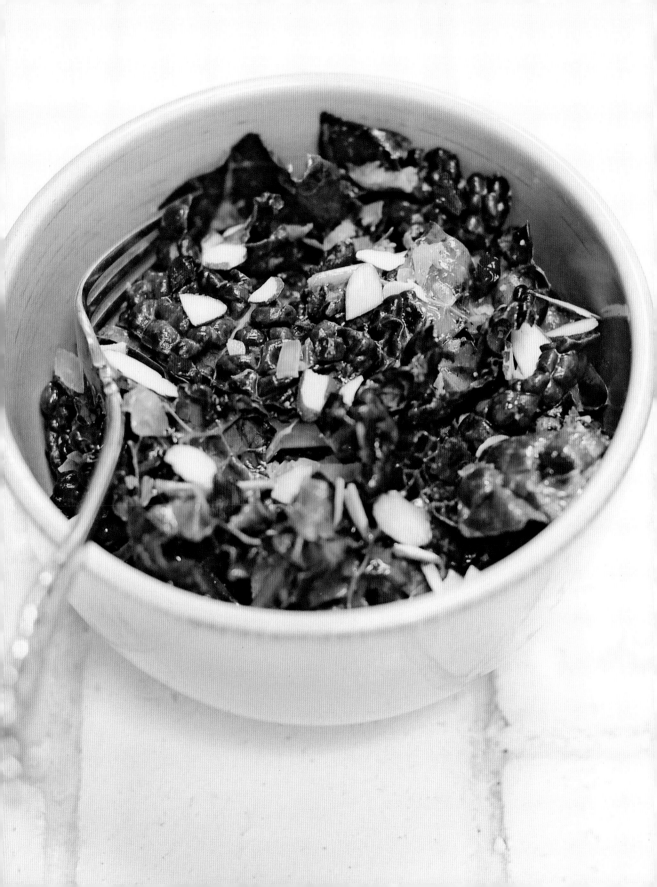

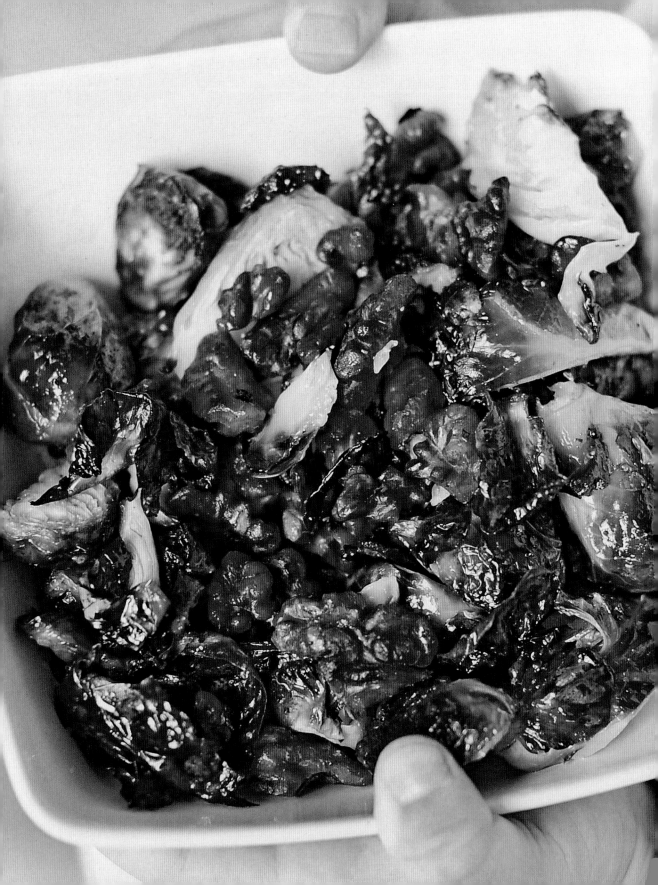

Zesty Walnut Brussels Sprouts

These brussels sprouts will please just about anyone's taste buds, thanks to a zing from the lemon juice. Be sure to make enough for leftovers, because they soak in flavor over time and are even better the next day.

½ cup (60 g) walnuts, chopped

1 pound (455 g) brussels sprouts, halved or quartered

2 to 3 tablespoons (27 to 40 g) coconut oil, melted

½ teaspoon salt

Ground black pepper, to taste

2 tablespoons (28 ml) extra-virgin olive oil

Juice from ½ of a lemon

—

Yield: 4 to 6 servings

NUTRITIONAL FACTS

Per serving, for 4 (5 oz, or 146 g): total carbs: 12.3 g; fiber: 5.2 g; net carbs: 7.1 g; protein: 5.8 g; fat: 22.2 g; calories: 252.

Per serving, for 6 (3.5 oz, or 98 g): total carbs: 8.2 g; fiber: 3.4 g; net carbs: 4.7 g; protein: 3.8 g; fat: 14.8 g; calories: 168.

Macronutrient ratio: calories from carbs: 18 percent; protein: 9 percent; fat: 74 percent.

Preheat the oven to 350°F (180°C, or gas mark 4). Scatter the walnuts on a baking sheet and bake for 10 minutes, or until toasted and fragrant. Set aside to cool.

Increase the oven to 400°F (200°C, or gas mark 6). Line a baking sheet with parchment paper.

In a medium bowl, toss together the brussels sprouts, coconut oil, salt, and pepper. Lay the sprouts out on the prepared baking sheet and roast for 35 minutes, or until fork-tender. Stir them halfway through baking to help them cook evenly.

Place the sprouts in a bowl and mix in the walnuts, olive oil, and lemon juice.

Store any leftovers in the fridge and then eat cool or warm briefly in the microwave or a pan.

Green Deviled Eggs & Bacon

These scrambled eggs with avocado and a side of bacon will become one of your favorite breakfasts. These are a great way to have that yummy, healthy breakfast as a fun, handheld snack.

4 slices nitrite-free bacon

4 eggs

1 ripe avocado

2 teaspoons (10 ml) hot sauce

Juice from ¼ lime

¼ teaspoon salt

Dash of garlic powder

Dash of smoked paprika for topping (optional)

—
Yield: 4 servings

NUTRITIONAL FACTS

Per serving (1 egg): total carbs: 3.6 g; fiber: 2.3 g; net carbs: 1.2 g; protein: 10 g; fat: 12.5 g; calories: 164.

Macronutrient ratio: calories from carbs: 9 percent; protein: 24 percent; fat: 68 percent.

Preheat the oven to 375°F (190°C, or gas mark 5). Line a baking sheet with aluminum foil. Set the bacon on a baking rack, if you have one, on the baking sheet and bake for 10 minutes on each side.

Meanwhile, place the eggs in a saucepan and cover them by 1 to 2 inches (2.5 to 5 cm) of cold water. Bring the water to a boil over high heat, and then remove the pan from the heat, cover, and let sit for 12 minutes. Pour out the hot water and replace with cold.

While the eggs and bacon are cooking, in a small bowl, combine the avocado, hot sauce, lime juice, salt, and garlic powder. Mix until fairly smooth.

When the eggs are cold, peel them and cut in half lengthwise. Gently remove the yolk (rinse if necessary, and place face-down on a paper towel to dry). Spoon the avocado mixture into the yolk hole. If you want to make it look pretty, cut about ¼ inch (6.5 mm) from the bottom corner of a sandwich bag, put the avocado mixture in, and squeeze it into the eggs.

Once the bacon has cooled, pat off the grease, crumble into bits, and add to the top of the avocado-filled eggs. Sprinkle paprika on top, if desired.

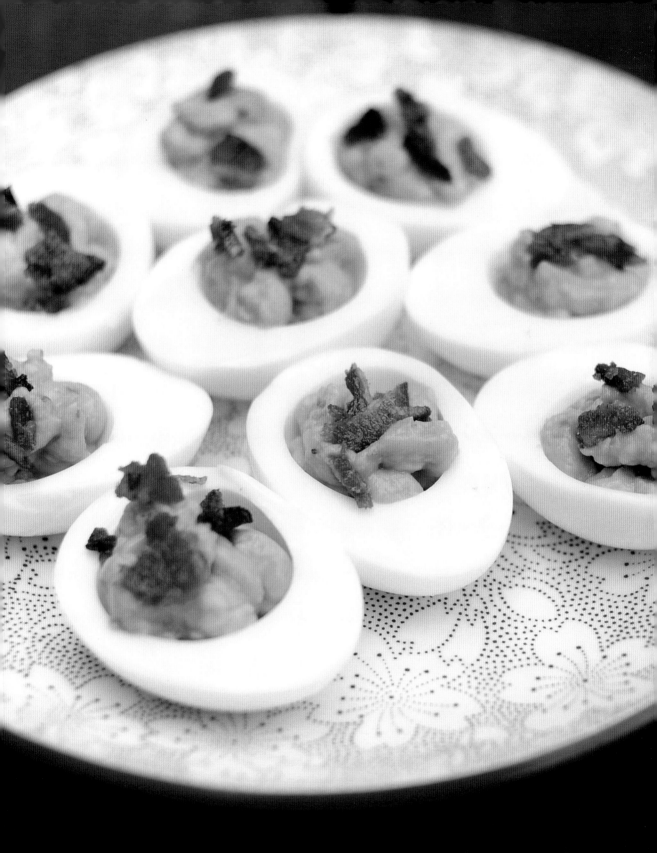

Prosciutto-Wrapped Asparagus

With just three simple ingredients, this supertasty snack is a great late afternoon treat. Serve it to your family and friends and before you know it, they'll all be gone . . . and that's a good thing!

1 pound (455 g) fresh asparagus

4 ounces (115 g) thinly sliced prosciutto

1 tablespoon (14 g) ghee or grass-fed butter

—

Yield: 4 servings

NUTRITIONAL FACTS

Per serving: total carbs: 2.4 g; fiber: 1.2 g; net carbs: 1.2 g; protein: 9.2 g; fat: 5.6 g; calories: 95.

Macronutrient ratio: calories from carbs: 10 percent; protein: 38 percent; fat: 52 percent.

Cut the bottom 2 inches (5 cm) off the asparagus. Then cut each slice of prosciutto in half lengthwise and individually wrap each piece around an asparagus spear.

In a large skillet over medium-high heat, melt the ghee. Add the wrapped asparagus and cook for about 2 minutes on each side, until the prosciutto is crispy. Reduce the heat to low and cook for about 10 minutes so the asparagus can steam.

Alternatively, you can roast them at 450°F (230°C, or gas mark 8) on a baking sheet. After you've wrapped the asparagus with prosciutto, brush them with melted ghee/butter, bake for 5 minutes on one side, flip, and bake for an additional 5 minutes.

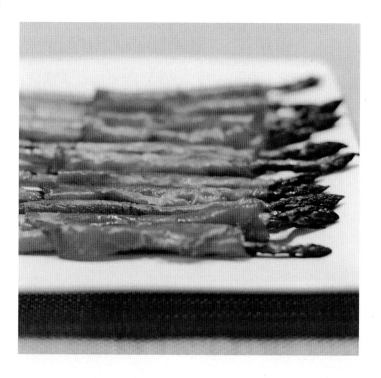

Cauliflower Hummus

Light and fluffy, this snack tastes even better than traditional hummus. It has all the wonderful flavors of a Greek snack, but without the difficult-to-digest legumes.

1 medium head of cauliflower (about 2 cups [200 g] florets)

⅓ cup (80 g) tahini

¼ cup (60 ml) fresh lemon juice

2 tablespoons (28 ml) extra-virgin olive oil

1 clove of garlic

¾ teaspoon salt

Ground black pepper, to taste

Dash of smoked paprika (optional)

—
Yield: 4 to 6 servings

NUTRITIONAL FACTS

Per serving, for 4 (6.75 oz, or 191 g): total carbs: 12.9 g; fiber: 3.9 g; net carbs: 9 g; protein: 6.4 g; fat: 18.1 g; calories: 220.

Per serving, for 6 (4.5 oz, or 127 g): total carbs: 8.6 g; fiber: 2.6 g; net carbs: 6 g; protein: 4.3 g; fat: 12 g; calories: 146.

Macronutrient ratio: calories from carbs: 22 percent; protein: 11 percent; fat: 68 percent.

Place a steamer basket in a medium pot and fill the pot with about 2 inches (5 cm) of water. If you don't have a basket, use a colander on top of your pot. Bring the water to a boil. Place the cauliflower florets in the steamer basket or colander. Cover and allow the florets to steam for 8 minutes, or until soft.

Transfer the cauliflower to a food processor. Add the tahini, lemon juice, olive oil, garlic, salt, and pepper. Blend until smooth. That's it! Dust with smoked paprika, if desired, before serving.

This hummus goes great with My Favorite Crunchy Crackers (page 78) or with any sliced raw veggies.

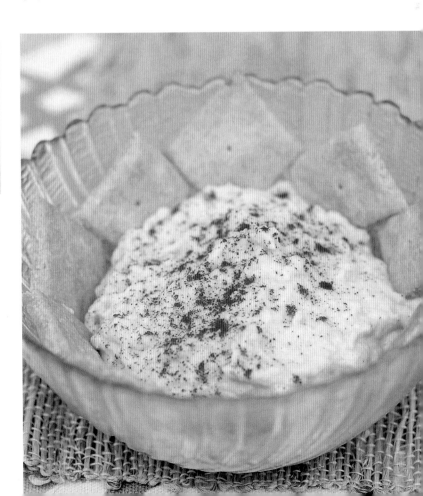

Roasted Red Pepper Dip

We all know how vitamin C is great for the common cold, but did you also know that it helps protect us from the harmful effects of stress? Vitamin C allows the body to quickly clear out cortisol, a primary stress hormone that increases sugars in the bloodstream. It just so happens that red peppers are the second highest plant source of vitamin C, containing almost 300 percent of our daily vitamin C intake. Mix all of that into a divine-tasting dip and you've got a superb snack!

1 cup (100 g) shelled walnuts

1 teaspoon smoked paprika

½ teaspoon onion powder

½ teaspoon salt

1 jar (12 ounces, or 340 g) roasted red peppers, drained

1 clove of garlic, minced

2 tablespoons (28 ml) extra-virgin olive oil

2 teaspoons lemon juice

—

Yield: about 4 servings

In a food processor, pulse the walnuts, paprika, onion powder, and salt until the walnuts are finely ground (like the consistency of hummus). Add the peppers, garlic, olive oil, and lemon juice and blend until completely smooth.

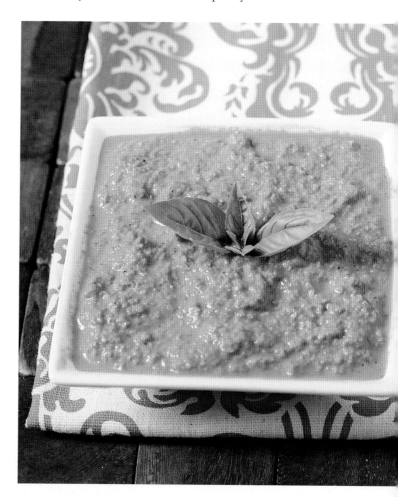

NUTRITIONAL FACTS

Per serving (3.5 oz, or 101 g): total carbs: 8.9 g; fiber: 4.3 g; net carbs: 4.6 g; protein: 4 g; fat: 23.4 g; calories: 250.

Macronutrient ratio: calories from carbs: 14 percent; protein: 6 percent; fat: 80 percent.

Flatbread "PB&J"

This supertasty roll-up will let you enjoy a sandwich-like snack without the guilt or worry of eating a high-carb, gluten-filled, high-glycemic bread. Great with sunflower seed butter and fresh, cut-up strawberries or the fruit of your choice, you'll never have to miss sandwich bread . . . or the peanut butter or jelly for that matter.

½ cup (56 g) coconut flour

2 tablespoons (16 g) psyllium husk powder

1 tablespoon (12 g) coconut palm sugar

1 teaspoon ground cinnamon

¼ cup (54 g) coconut oil

1 cup (235 ml) boiling water

⅓ cup (75 g) sunflower seed butter

10 strawberries, thinly sliced

—
Yield: 5 sandwiches

NUTRITIONAL FACTS

Per sandwich: total carbs: 19.8 g; fiber: 9.3 g; net carbs: 10.5 g; protein: 4.7 g; fat: 21.9 g; calories: 286.

Macronutrient ratio: calories from carbs: 27 percent; protein: 6 percent; fat: 67 percent.

Preheat the oven to 375°F (190°C, or gas mark 5). Line a baking sheet with parchment paper. In a medium bowl, mix together the coconut flour, psyllium husk powder, coconut palm sugar, and cinnamon. Add the coconut oil and hot water and stir it all together.

Spread the dough out on the lined baking sheet. With a rolling pin or glass, flatten out the dough as evenly as you can so it's about ½ inch (1.5 cm) thick. Bake 15 minutes, or until a toothpick inserted in the middle comes out clean. Then move to a cooling rack and allow to cool to room temperature.

Once the dough is cool, spread the sunflower seed butter and strawberries (or whatever fruit you would like). Then carefully roll the "bread" and slice, with a pizza cutter or knife, into 3 inch (7.5 cm) pieces.

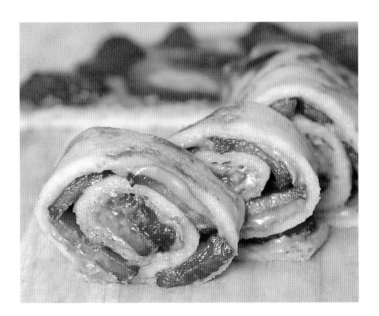

Pork Belly Fat Bombs

If you're lucky enough to have leftover pork belly, use it to make these snack-size fat bombs. They're meaty and filling and, because they're laced with mustard and horseradish, they also pack quite a kick!

5.3 ounces (150 g) cooked pork belly (see Note)

6 pancetta slices or 3 bacon slices (3.2 ounces, or 90 g), cut in half widthwise

¼ cup (55 g/1.9 oz) mayonnaise, preferably homemade

1 tablespoon (15 g/0.5 oz) Dijon mustard

1 tablespoon (15 g/0.5 oz) grated fresh horseradish

Salt and pepper, to taste

Crispy lettuce leaves, for serving (optional)

—
Yield: 6 servings

NUTRITIONAL FACTS

Per serving: total carbs: 0.5 g; fiber: 0.2 g; net carbs: 0.3 g; protein: 5.8 g; fat: 26.4 g; energy: 263 kcal.

Macronutrient ratio: calories from carbs: 1 percent; protein: 9 percent; fat: 90 percent.

Preheat the oven to 375°F (190°C, or gas mark 5). Line a baking sheet with parchment paper. Lay the bacon slices flat on the parchment, leaving enough space between so they don't overlap. Place the sheet in the oven and cook for 10 to 15 minutes, or until crispy. The exact amount of cooking time depends on the thickness of the bacon slices. Remove from the oven and set aside to cool. Pour the bacon grease into a glass container and reserve for another use, such as frying eggs. When cool enough to handle, crumble the bacon into a dish and set aside.

Shred the pork belly in a bowl. Mix in the mayonnaise, mustard, and horseradish. Season with salt and pepper. Divide the mixture into six mounds. Top with the crumbled bacon and serve on top of crispy lettuce leaves (if using). Enjoy immediately or refrigerate in an airtight container for up to 5 days.

NOTE:

If you need to cook the pork belly, preheat the oven to 400°F (200°C, or gas mark 6). Using a sharp knife, score the pork skin down to the meat. Make the cuts close together and try not to cut the meat. Place it in a deep roasting pan and into the preheated oven. Cook for 30 minutes. Reduce the temperature to 325°F (160°C, or gas mark 3), and cook for 1 hour, 30 minutes more. Finally, increase the temperature to 425°F (220°C, or gas mark 7), and cook for another 30 minutes. Remove from the oven and set aside to cool at room temperature.

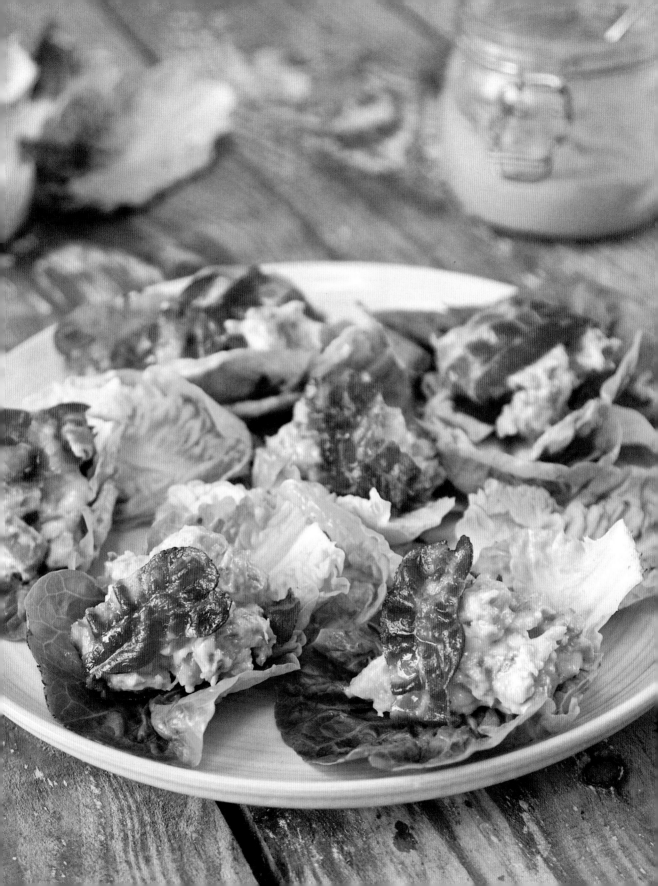

N'Oatmeal Cookies

You might remember the irresistible, old-fashioned oatmeal raisin cookies made with Crisco, white flour, sugar, and oats. Fast-forward to these N'Oatmeal Cookies—healthwise, the antithesis of the old-fashioned variety, but tastewise, equally as good.

2 cups (200 g) almond meal

½ cup (96 g) coconut palm sugar

2 tablespoons (16 g) arrowroot powder

1 tablespoon (7 g) ground cinnamon

1 teaspoon salt

¾ teaspoon baking soda

4 eggs, room temperature

½ cup (112 g) grass-fed butter, melted

¼ cup (85 g) maple syrup

1 teaspoon vanilla extract

½ cup (50 g) raw walnuts, roughly chopped

½ cup (50 g) raw pecans, roughly chopped

½ cup (73 g) raw almonds, roughly chopped

½ cup (75 g) raisins

—
Yield: about 18 cookies

Preheat the oven to 350°F (180°C, or gas mark 4). Line a baking sheet with parchment paper.

In a small bowl, mix together the almond meal, coconut palm sugar, arrowroot, cinnamon, salt, and baking soda. In a medium bowl, beat the eggs and then mix in the butter, maple syrup, and vanilla. Pour the dry ingredients into the wet and combine well. Fold in the walnuts, pecans, almonds, and raisins.

Use your hands or a tablespoon to shape the dough into 2½ inch (6.5 cm) cookies. Bake for 8 to 10 minutes, or until set.

NUTRITIONAL FACTS

Per cookie: total carbs: 17.3 g; fiber: 2.6 g; net carbs: 14.7 g; protein: 5.7 g; fat: 18.1 g; calories: 243.

Macronutrient ratio: calories from carbs: 27 percent; protein: 9 percent; fat: 64 percent.

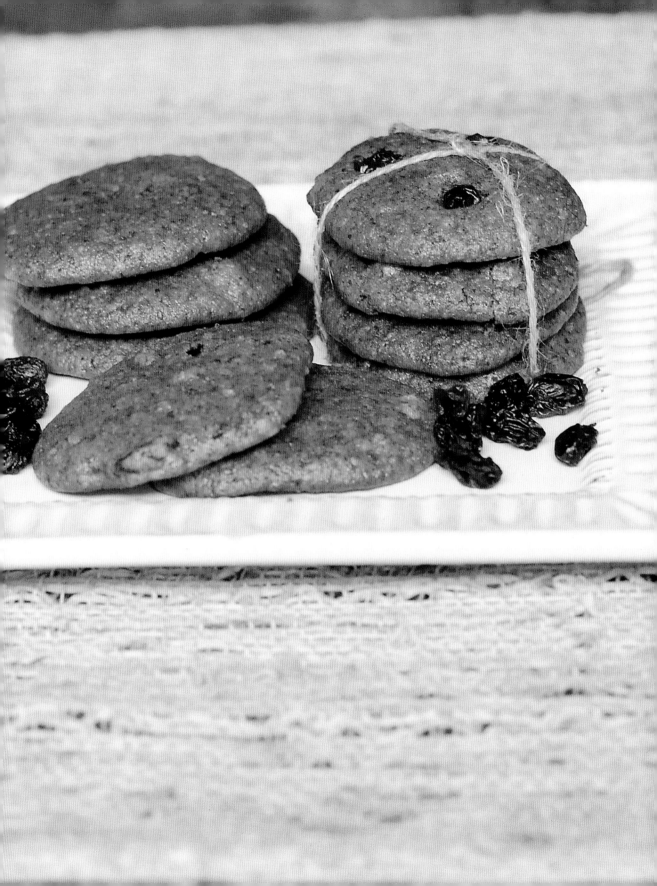

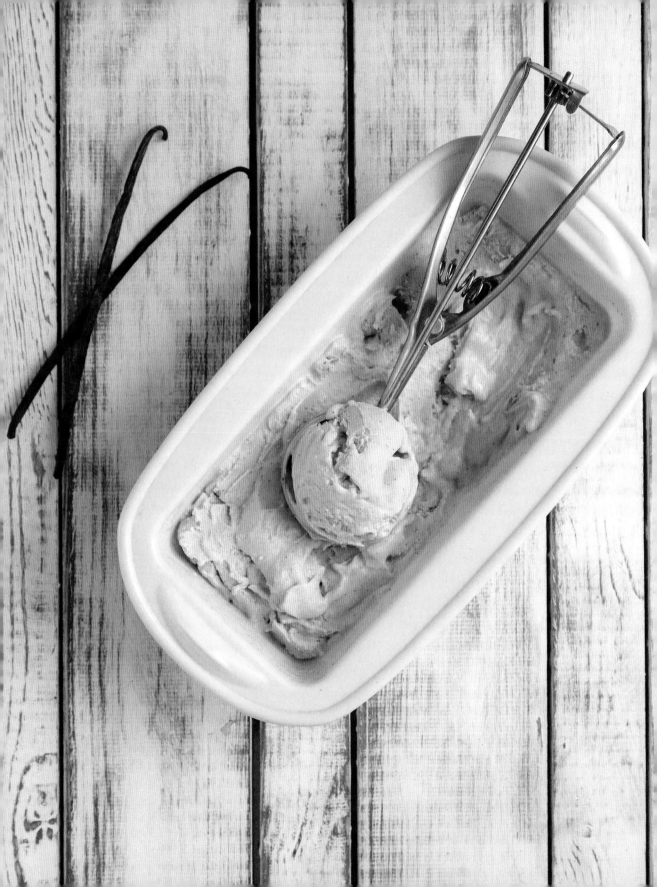

Vanilla-Keto Ice Cream

This low-carb ice cream is a scoopable fat bomb—and it's so ridiculously rich and creamy that you'll mistake it for frozen vanilla custard.

1½ cups (360 g/12.7 oz) creamed coconut milk

6 large egg yolks

2 large eggs

¼ cup (40 g/1.4 oz) erythritol or Swerve, powdered

¼ cup (60 ml /2 fl oz) MCT oil

2 teaspoons sugar-free vanilla extract or 1 teaspoon vanilla powder

Few drops liquid stevia, to taste (optional)

—

Yield: 8 servings/scoops

NUTRITIONAL FACTS

Per serving (1 scoop [⅓ cup/85 g/ 3 oz]): total carbs: 3.9 g; fiber: 1 g; net carbs: 2.9 g; protein: 5.2 g; fat: 27.1 g; energy: 270 kcal.

Macronutrient ratio: calories from carbs: 4 percent; protein: 8 percent; fat: 88 percent.

Make the creamed coconut milk a day ahead (see below for instructions).

In a food processor, combine the creamed coconut milk, egg yolks, eggs, erythritol, MCT oil, and vanilla. Pulse until smooth and creamy. If you want a sweeter taste, add the stevia and pulse again.

Pour the mixture into an ice cream maker and process according to the manufacturer's instructions. Once the ice cream is churned, freeze for about 30 minutes before serving. Keep frozen for up to 3 months.

HOW TO MAKE CREAMED COCONUT MILK: Creamed coconut milk or coconut cream is the fatty part of coconut milk that has been separated from the watery part. If a recipe calls for creamed coconut milk, make it a day ahead. To "cream" coconut milk, simply place the can in the refrigerator overnight. The next day, open the can, spoon out the solidified coconut milk, and discard the liquids. Do not shake the can before opening. One 14 ounce (400 g)-can will yield about 7 ounces (200 g) of coconut cream.

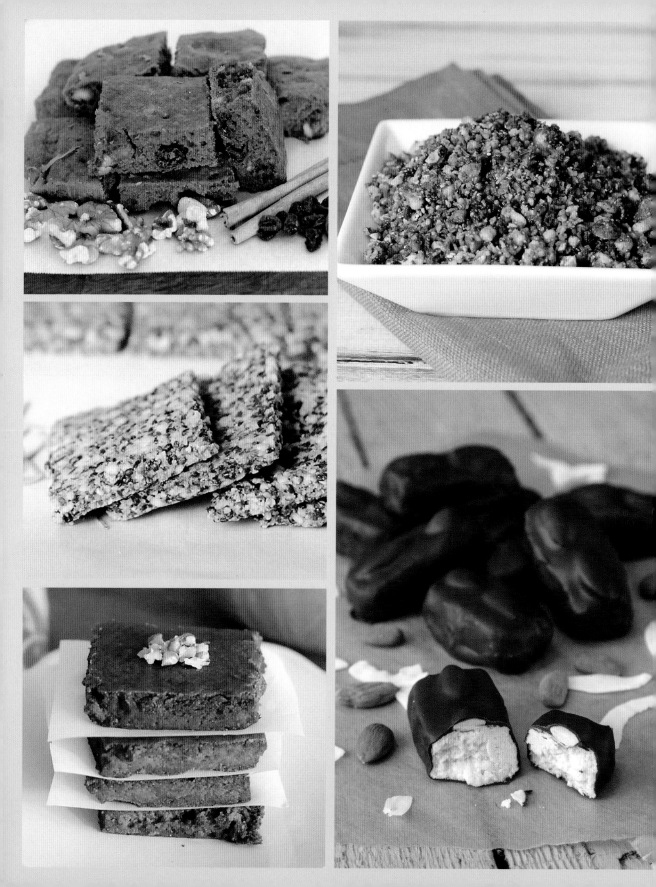

4

ON-THE-GO SNACKS: Fun and Convenient for Commutes, Carpools, and Road Trips

We spend a great deal of our lives in the car. It's a necessary part of life. Whether you are going to work, carpooling to a child's activity, or heading out on a fun road trip, choosing the right snacks can be challenging. What can you bring that is fun, portable, tasty, easy to eat, keeps well, and of course, actually good for you?

Unfortunately, many prepackaged snacks are laden with preservatives and food coloring that, according to recent research by the UK's government-sponsored Food Commission, can increase temper tantrums and irritable behavior.

Fortunately for you, this chapter contains delicious snacks that are both fun and easy to eat—no spoon feeding or face wiping of little ones. They're made with no artificial colors, additives, or processed sugar. Even better, because they're low-glycemic, they will keep blood sugar levels stable.

Moreover, all these snacks fit neatly into sandwich bags or small storage containers, making them superportable.

Crispy Maple Granola 73

Mini Zucchini Muffins 74

Chocolate Chip Muffins 77

Favorite Crackers 78

Cinnamon Raisin Bars 80

Chile-Lime Peanuts 81

Pumpkin Bars 82

"Peanut Butter" Cookies 84

Blonde Snack Bars 86

Almond Bliss Bars 89

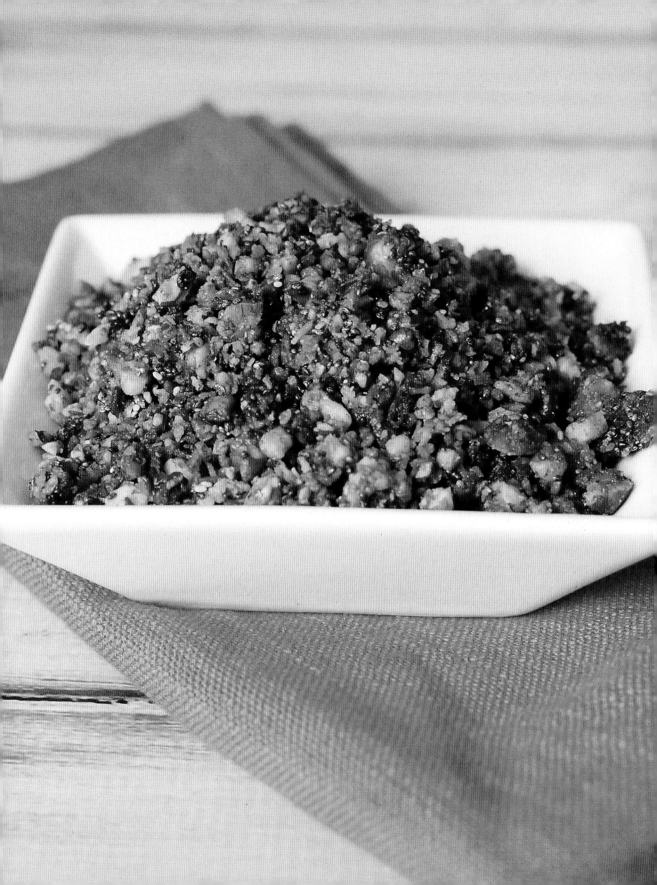

Crispy Maple Granola

There is something about a sweet, salty, crunchy, and buttery treat all wrapped into one snack that is amazing. Add to that the health benefits of the grass-fed butter, which include immune-boosting, cancer-fighting, fat-burning nutrients. Also loaded with fiber, omega-3s, and other healthy fats, this snack is great for a car ride as it will keep you satiated a long time, or even at home with berries and almond or coconut milk.

¾ cup (75 g) raw pecans

½ cup (73 g) raw almonds

½ cup (50 g) raw walnuts

¾ cup (60 g) unsweetened shredded coconut

3 tablespoons (30 g) chia seeds

¼ cup (85 g) maple syrup

2½ tablespoons (35 g) grass-fed butter

1½ teaspoons vanilla extract

¼ teaspoon salt

—
Yield: 3 cups (366 g)

Preheat the oven to 325°F (170°C, or gas mark 3). Line a baking sheet with parchment paper.

In a food processor, pulse the pecans, almonds, and walnuts into small pieces. Pour into a medium bowl with the shredded coconut and chia seeds; toss to combine. In a small saucepan, over medium-low heat, cook the maple syrup, butter, vanilla, and salt until it starts to bubble. Pour the liquid mixture over the nuts, coconut, and seeds. Mix well.

Spread onto the prepared baking sheet so it's not overlapping too much. Bake for 20 minutes, or until it starts to turn golden brown, tossing a couple of times so it cooks evenly. Once it comes out and starts to cool, it will get crunchier.

NUTRITIONAL FACTS

Per ¼-cup serving (1 oz, or 34 g): total carbs: 9.5 g; fiber: 3 g; net carbs: 6.5 g; protein: 3.2 g; fat: 16.8 g; calories: 194.

Macronutrient ratio: calories from carbs: 19 percent; protein: 6 percent; fat: 75 percent.

Mini Zucchini Muffins

These fun, supertasty, and easy-to-eat mini muffins are like little shots of omega-3s for your brain. Studies have shown omega-3s can increase happiness and relaxation. Who couldn't use a little more of that while on the road?

1 cup (112 g) almond flour

1 cup (128 g) flaxseed meal

⅓ cup (64 g) coconut palm sugar

1½ teaspoons ground cinnamon

½ teaspoon salt

½ teaspoon baking soda

2 eggs

¼ cup (55 g) grass-fed butter, melted

½ cup (60 g) chopped raw walnuts

⅓ cup (50 g) currants or raisins

1 cup (124 g) peeled and grated zucchini (about 2 medium)

—
Yield: 32 mini muffins

Preheat the oven to 350°F (180°C, or gas mark 4). Grease a mini-muffin pan.

In a medium bowl, mix the almond flour, flaxseed meal, coconut palm sugar, cinnamon, salt, and baking soda. In a small bowl, beat the eggs, and then add the melted butter, walnuts, and raisins. Add the wet ingredients to the dry and mix until well blended. Then mix in the zucchini until combined.

Scoop the batter into the prepared muffin cups about they are three-quarters full. Bake for 25 minutes, or until a toothpick inserted in the middle of a muffin comes out clean.

NUTRITIONAL FACTS

Per muffin: total carbs: 5.6 g; fiber: 1.6 g; net carbs: 3.9 g; protein: 2.3 g; fat: 5.4 g; calories: 75.

Macronutrient ratio: calories from carbs: 28 percent; protein: 11 percent; fat: 61 percent.

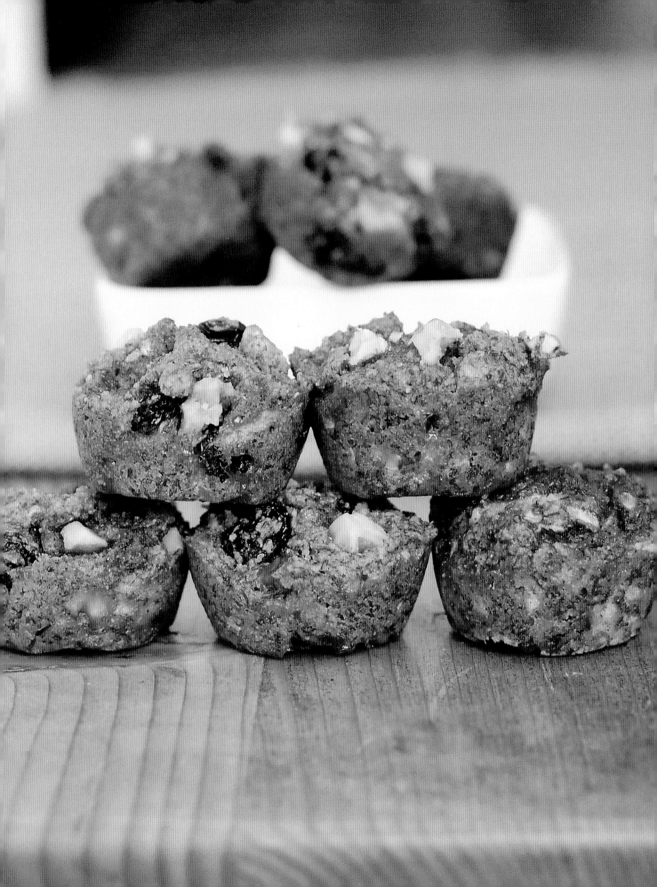

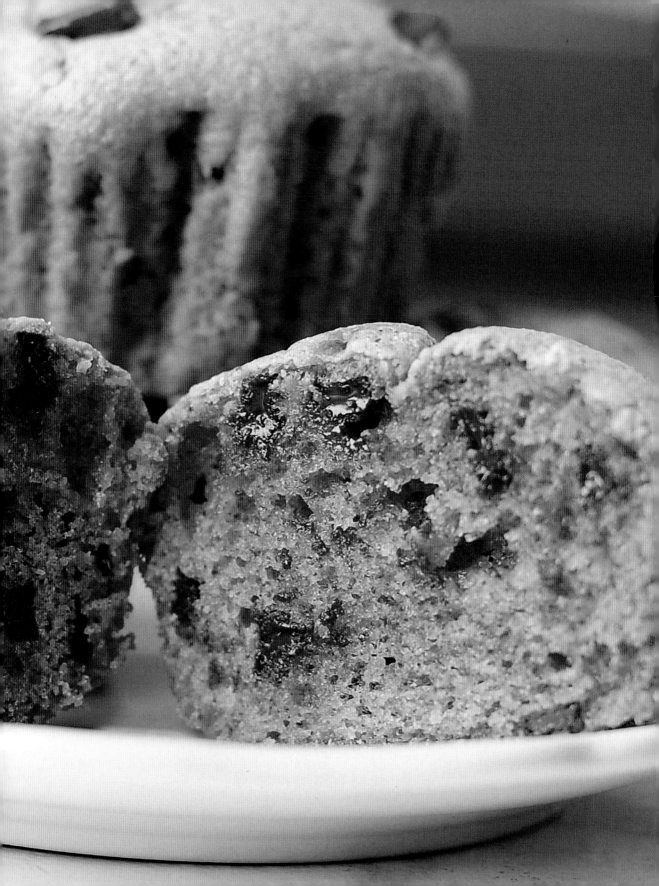

Chocolate Chip Muffins

These moist and delicious little snacks will not only satisfy your taste buds but will keep you feeling full thanks to an abundance of healthy fats. Because they are made with low-glycemic sweeteners and a little caffeine (thank you, chocolate), these muffins will recharge your batteries—without the big sugar spike and fall associated with most sweet snacks. Try to set your eggs out ahead of time so they can warm to room temperature. Otherwise, the chill from the eggs will solidify the coconut oil and can make the batter clumpy.

3 eggs, room temperature

½ teaspoon vanilla extract

1 cup (260 g) almond butter

1 cup (112 g) almond flour

½ cup (96 g) coconut palm sugar

⅓ cup (72 g) coconut oil, melted

½ teaspoon baking soda

¼ teaspoon salt

½ cup (88 g) dark chocolate chips

—

Yield: 12 muffins

Preheat the oven to 350°F (180°C, or gas mark 4). Line a 12-cup muffin pan with silicone or paper muffin liners, or grease the cups.

In a small bowl, beat the eggs and then add the vanilla. In a medium bowl, mix together the almond butter, almond flour, coconut palm sugar, coconut oil, baking soda, and salt. Add the egg mixture and stir until well combined. Fold in the chocolate chips.

Pour the batter into the prepared muffin cups until about two-thirds full. Bake for 20 minutes, or until a toothpick inserted in the middle of a muffin comes out clean. Cool slightly before removing muffins from pan.

NUTRITIONAL FACTS

Per muffin: total carbs: 20.1 g; fiber: 3.2 g; net carbs: 16.3 g; protein: 8.7 g; fat: 26.7 g; calories: 333.

Macronutrient ratio: calories from carbs: 23 percent; protein: 10 percent; fat: 68 percent.

Favorite Crackers

There is no better name for this cracker. Low-glycemic and full of protein, with good fats including lots of omega-3s, this easy-to-eat snack is ideal for in the car, or anywhere else for that matter.

1 cup (112 g) almond flour

½ cup (64 g) flaxseed meal

½ cup (92 g) chia seeds

1¼ teaspoons (7.5 g) salt

2 teaspoons (3 g) Italian seasoning

1 teaspoon garlic powder

1 egg

2 tablespoons (28 ml) extra-virgin olive oil

—

Yield: about 50 crackers

NUTRITIONAL FACTS

Per cracker (¼ oz, or 7 g): total carbs: 1.6 g; fiber: 1.1 g; net carbs: 0.5 g; protein: 1.1 g; fat: 2.6 g; calories: 32.

Macronutrient ratio: calories from carbs: 19 percent; protein: 13 percent; fat: 68 percent.

Preheat the oven to 350°F (180°C, or gas mark 4).

In a medium bowl, combine the almond flour, flaxseed meal, chia seeds, salt, Italian seasoning, garlic powder, and mix well. Add the egg and olive oil and stir until a dough forms.

Place half of the dough on a piece of parchment paper. Top with another piece of parchment paper and roll with rolling pin to about ⅛ inch (3 mm) thick. Remove the top piece of parchment. With a pizza cutter, score individual crackers into squares. Transfer the dough and bottom piece of parchment to a baking sheet. Bake for 8 minutes, or until they start to turn brown. Then turn off the heat and let them sit in the oven for another 10 minutes or so.

Once those are done, you can lay out the second batch on the prepared baking sheet and begin baking them. You can also bake them on two baking sheets, one on each rack in the oven; just shuffle the baking sheets halfway through the bake time.

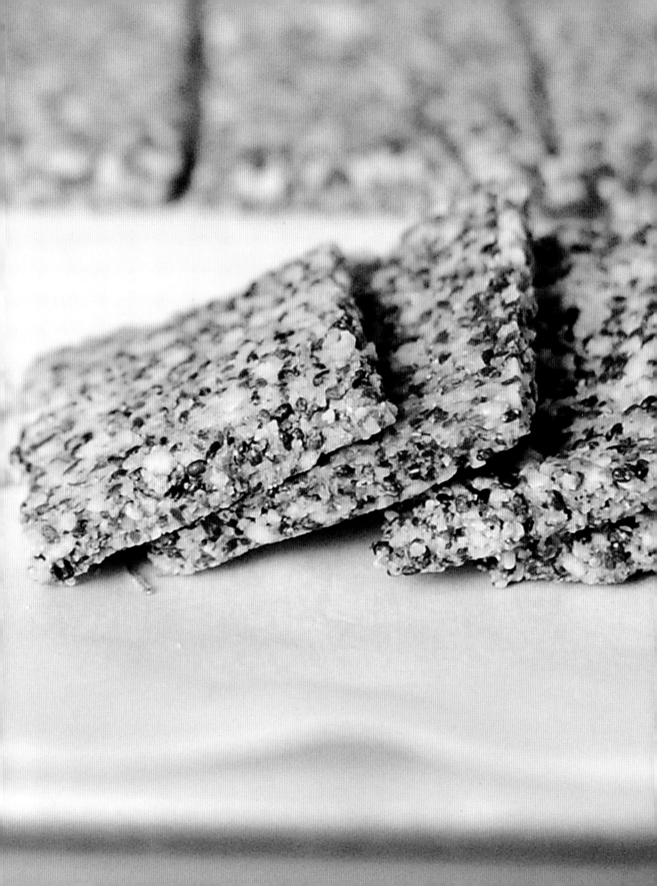

Cinnamon Raisin Bars

Reminiscent of old-school cinnamon raisin bread, this delicious and easy-to-eat snack is perfect for the car. It can also be made nut-free by substituting the almond butter with a sunflower seed butter and leaving out the walnuts (or substituting with dark chocolate chips).

4 eggs

1 cup (260 g) almond butter or sunflower seed butter

⅓ cup (115 g) maple syrup

2 tablespoons (28 g) grass-fed butter, melted

2 tablespoons (24 g) coconut palm sugar

2 tablespoons (14 g) ground cinnamon

1 teaspoon vanilla extract

½ teaspoon baking soda

½ teaspoon salt

¼ cup (35 g) raisins or currants

¼ cup (25 g) walnuts (optional)

—
Yield: 16 bars

Preheat the oven to 325°F (170°C, or gas mark 3). Grease an 8 x 8-inch (20 x 20-cm) baking dish with coconut oil or palm shortening.

In a large bowl, combine the eggs, almond butter, maple syrup, butter, coconut palm sugar, cinnamon, vanilla, baking soda, and salt and stir until smooth. Fold in the raisins and walnuts, if using. Pour the batter into the prepared baking dish and move the dish around to ensure the batter is even. Bake for 25 minutes, or until a toothpick inserted in the middle of the bars comes out clean. Allow to cool for 30 minutes before cutting into bars and enjoying.

NUTRITIONAL FACTS

Per serving, w/o walnuts: total carbs: 11.9 g; fiber: 2.3 g; net carbs: 9.7 g; protein: 5.1 g; fat: 11.6 g; calories: 163.

Macronutrient ratio: calories from carbs: 28 percent; protein: 12 percent; fat: 60 percent.

Per serving, w/ walnuts: total carbs: 12.2 g; fiber: 2.4 g; net carbs: 9.8 g; protein: 5.3 g; fat: 12.6 g; calories: 174.

Macronutrient ratio: calories from carbs: 26 percent; protein: 12 percent; fat: 62 percent.

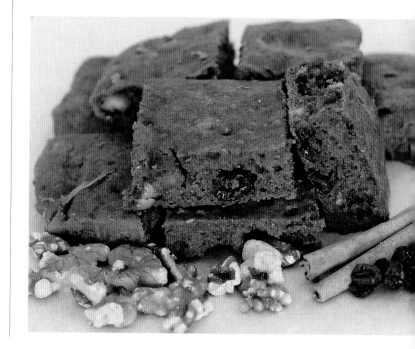

Chile-Lime Peanuts

Crunchy, a little spicy, with a Southwestern kick, these are supertasty—and superportable!

12 ounces (340 g) raw, shelled peanuts

1½ tablespoons (21 g) coconut oil, melted

1 tablespoon (15 ml) lime juice

½ teaspoon pure ground chile powder

½ teaspoon paprika (Smoked paprika is great, but use what you have.)

⅛ teaspoon cayenne pepper

Salt, to taste

—
Yield: 12 servings

NUTRITIONAL FACTS

Per serving (1 oz, or 32 g): total carbs: 4.8 g; fiber: 2.5 g; net carbs: 2.3 g; protein: 7.4 g; fat: 15.7 g; calories: 177.

Macronutrient ratio: calories from carbs: 10 percent; protein: 16 percent; fat: 74 percent.

Preheat the oven to 350°F (180°C, or gas mark 4). Line a jelly roll pan with aluminum foil.

Dump the peanuts onto the pan.

In a small dish, mix together the coconut oil, lime juice, chile powder, paprika, and cayenne.

Slowly pour the seasoning mixture over the peanuts, stirring the nuts constantly. Make sure they're all evenly coated.

Put them in the oven and set the timer for 5 minutes. When it beeps, remove and stir them again and return to the oven for another 5 minutes. Stir again, return to the oven, and give them a final 5 minutes.

Sprinkle with salt and let cool. Store in a tightly lidded container.

NOTE:

Look around your grocery stores for peanuts in bulk, which are often cheaper than the packaged variety.

Pumpkin Bars

These savory treats are perfectly sweetened. With a whole cup of pumpkin in the mix, this snack is full of fiber to keep you full, as well as vitamin A and iron to help keep your immune system strong.

1 cup (245 g) pumpkin purée

½ cup (130 g) almond butter

⅓ cup (64 g) coconut palm sugar

1 tablespoon (7 g) coconut flour

1 tablespoon (7 g) pumpkin pie spice

1 tablespoon (20 g) maple syrup

½ teaspoon vanilla extract

2 eggs

¼ teaspoon baking soda

⅛ teaspoon salt

Handful of walnuts, chopped (optional)

—

Yield: 12 bars

Preheat the oven to 350°F (180°C, or gas mark 4). Grease an 8 x 8-inch (20 x 20-cm) baking dish.

In a large bowl (or food processor), mix together the pumpkin purée, almond butter, palm sugar, coconut flour, pumpkin pie spice, maple syrup, vanilla, eggs, baking soda, and salt until well blended. Pour the mixture into the prepared baking dish. Bake for about 40 minutes, or until a toothpick inserted in the middle comes out clean. Allow to cool for about 30 minutes and then eat as is or top with chopped walnuts.

NUTRITIONAL FACTS

Per bar: total carbs: 10.9 g; fiber: 2 g; net carbs: 8.9 g; protein: 3.6 g; fat: 6.9 g; calories: 113.

Macronutrient ratio: calories from carbs: 36 percent; protein: 12 percent; fat: 52 percent.

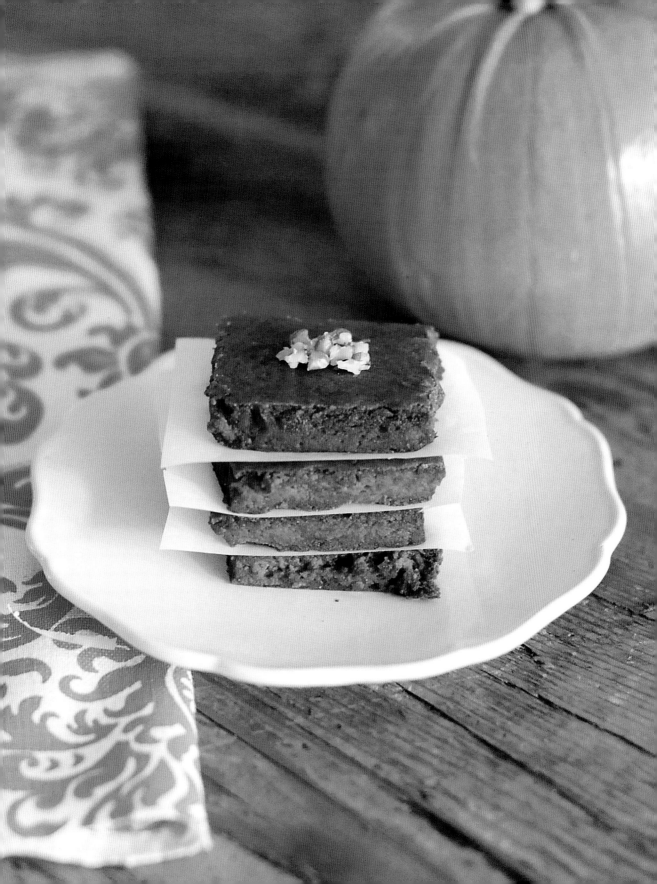

"Peanut Butter" Cookies

Sunflower seeds have a similar makeup to that of peanuts. When it comes to oil, protein, and carbohydrate contents, they're pretty close. The taste of these cookies is as close as you can get to a peanut butter cookie, and just as mouthwatering, but without the peanuts. Sunflower seeds also are considered to be one of the best whole-food sources of vitamin E, which helps protect brain cells and lowers the risk for chronic diseases. So now you have an excuse to eat even more of this rich, delectable treat!

2 cups (520 g) sunflower seed butter (16-ounce jar)

1 cup (192 g) coconut palm sugar

1 tablespoon (15 ml) vanilla extract

¼ teaspoon salt

—

Yield: about 24 cookies

NUTRITIONAL FACTS

Per cookie: total carbs: 13 g; fiber: 1.2 g; net carbs: 11.8 g; protein: 3.7 g; fat: 11.8 g; calories: 163.

Macronutrient ratio: calories from carbs: 30 percent; protein: 9 percent; fat: 61 percent.

Preheat the oven to 350°F (180°C, or gas mark 4). Line a baking sheet with parchment paper.

In a medium bowl, mix together the sunflower seed butter, coconut palm sugar, vanilla extract, and salt and stir until well combined. Form golf ball–size pieces of dough and set on the prepared baking sheet. (Make sure the cookies have about 1 inch [2.5 cm] between them. You may have to use two baking sheets or bake in two batches.) Press the dough down to make the cookies a little flat and then use a fork to press a crisscross pattern onto them. Bake for 10 minutes, or until a toothpick inserted in the middle of a cookie comes out clean. (They will not turn brown on top like traditional peanut butter cookies.) Enjoy!

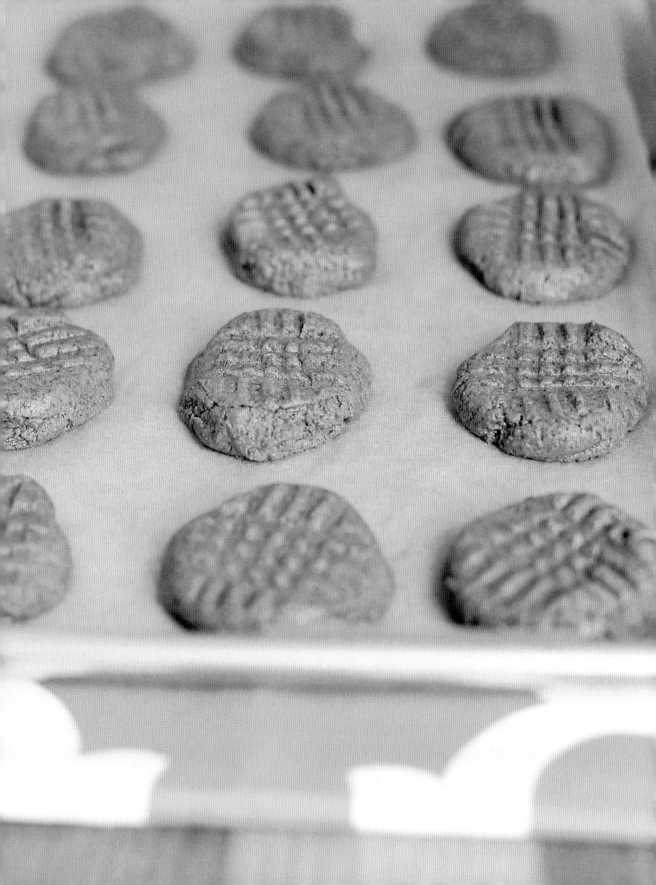

Blonde Snack Bars

These moist, fluffy, and delicious bars taste like dessert! Because they are high in protein, have lots of healthy fat from the almond butter, and contain only low-glycemic sugars, they won't cause blood sugar swings or ramp up cravings like most traditional sweets or packaged snacks would.

2 cups (520 g) almond butter

6 eggs

1 cup (192 g) coconut palm sugar

4 teaspoons (20 ml) vanilla extract

1 teaspoon salt

1 teaspoon baking soda

1 cup (175 g) dark chocolate chips

—

Yield: 24 bars

Preheat the oven to 325°F (170°C, or gas mark 3). Grease a 9 x 13 inch (23 x 33 cm) baking dish or pan.

In a medium bowl, mix together the almond butter, eggs, coconut palm sugar, vanilla, salt, and baking soda. Fold in the chocolate chips. Spread the batter into the prepared dish and bake for 45 to 50 minutes, until a toothpick inserted in the middle comes out clean. Allow to cool for 10 minutes before cutting into bars.

To make these nut-free, you can use sunflower seed butter, but be aware that as the bars cool, the insides will turn green due to a chemical reaction with the baking soda. They are still totally fine and good to eat. Might be a great snack for St. Patrick's Day!

NUTRITIONAL FACTS

Per bar: total carbs: 18.2 g; fiber: 2.2 g; net carbs: 15.3 g; protein: 6.7 g; fat: 16.1 g; calories: 228.

Macronutrient ratio: calories from carbs: 30 percent; protein: 11 percent; fat: 59 percent.

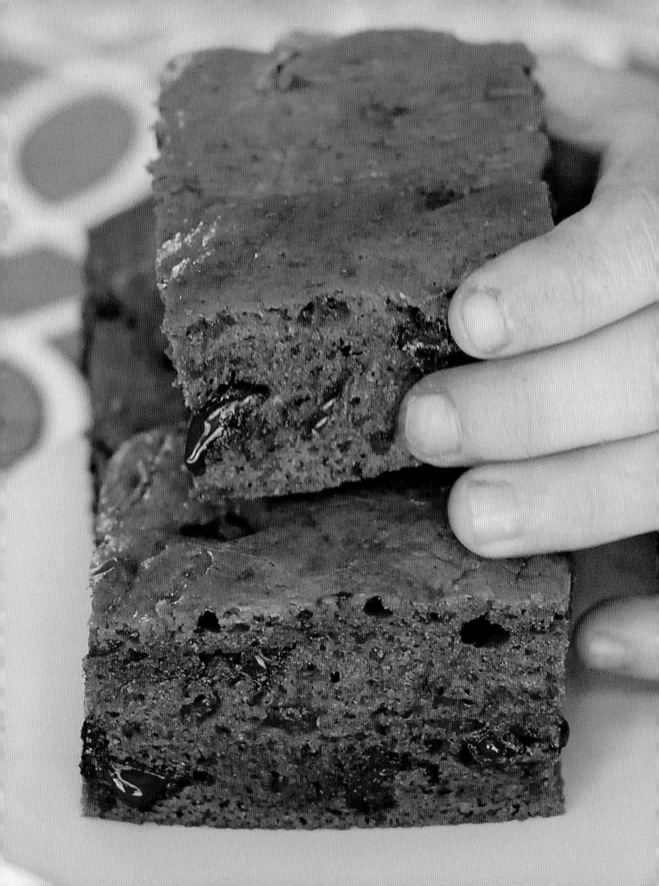

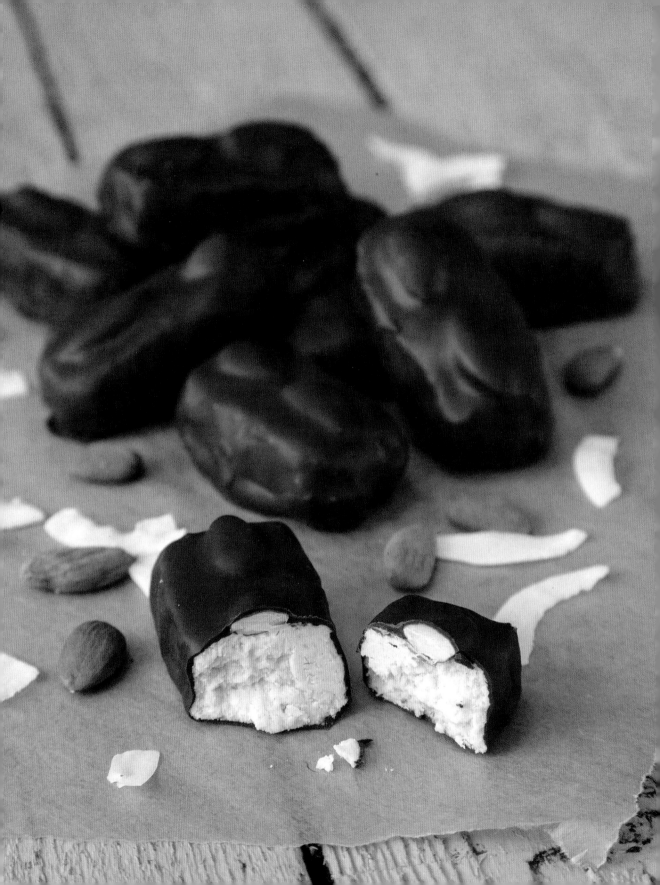

Almond Bliss Bars

Chocolate and coconut: it's like the perfect island wedding. Add almonds, and it's the perfect love triangle! These sugar-free bars are absolutely irresistible and make a great post-workout snack.

FOR BARS:

½ cup (120 g/4.2 oz) creamed coconut milk

1½ cups (112 g/4 oz) unsweetened shredded coconut

¼ cup (55 g/1.9 oz) coconut oil, at room temperature

2 tablespoons (20 g/0.7 oz) erythritol or Swerve, powdered

2 teaspoons sugar-free vanilla extract or 1 teaspoon vanilla powder

Pinch salt

Few drops liquid stevia, to taste (optional)

20 whole almonds (24 g/0.8 oz)

FOR COATING (OR USE ANY OF THE HOMEMADE DARK CHOCOLATE RECIPES [PAGE 24]):

2 ounces (56 g) extra-dark 90 percent chocolate

0.8 ounces (24 g) cacao butter

—
Yield: 10 servings

TO MAKE CREAMED COCONUT MILK, follow the instructions on page 69.

TO MAKE THE BARS: In a mixing bowl, stir together the creamed coconut milk, shredded coconut, coconut oil, erythritol, vanilla, and salt. If you want a sweeter taste, add the stevia and mix again. Use your hands to form the mixture into 10 small bars, about 1 ounce/(32 g) each, and place them on a parchment-lined tray. Top each bar with 2 almonds. Freeze for about 30 minutes.

TO MAKE THE COATING: Melt the dark chocolate in a double boiler, or heat-proof bowl placed over a small saucepan filled with 1 cup of water, over medium heat. Remove from the heat and set aside to cool.

Gently pierce each bar with a toothpick or a fork. Working one at a time, hold each bar over the melted dark chocolate and spoon the chocolate over it to coat completely. Turn the stick as you work until the coating is solidified. Place the coated bars on a parchment-lined tray and drizzle any remaining coating over them.

Refrigerate the coated bars for at least 15 minutes to harden. Keep refrigerated for up to 1 week or freeze for up to 3 months.

NUTRITIONAL FACTS

Per serving (1 bar): total carbs: 5.3 g; fiber: 2.8 g; net carbs: 2.5 g; protein: 3.8 g; fat: 17.8 g; energy: 193 kcal.

Macronutrient ratio: calories from carbs: 5 percent; protein: 8 percent; fat: 87 percent.

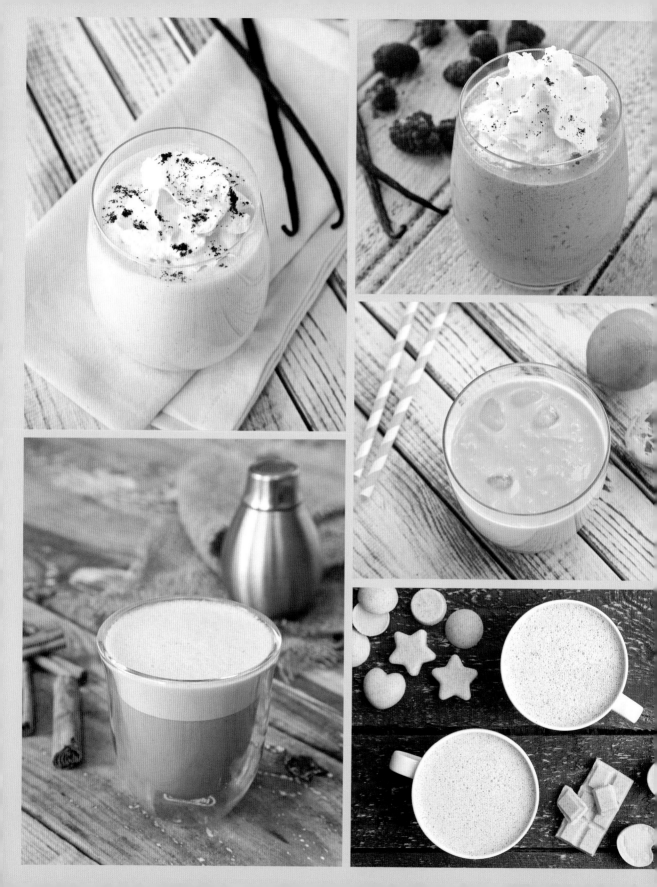

5

SIPPABLE SNACKS: Blissful Beverages for Any Time of Day

Low-carb snacks come in many different shapes and sizes—including refreshing smoothies and satisfying hot beverages. Plenty of the beverages in this chapter are nutritious enough to count as filling snacks. Most are high in healthy fats, which help you stay fuller longer, so they're also perfect for breakfasts or light lunches. And they're quick to prepare—most of the recipes in this chapter take only a few minutes to whip up.

Creamy Dark Hot Chocolate 93

Creamy White Hot Chocolate 94

Creamy Keto Coffee 97

Coconut-Vanilla Coffee 98

Cococcino 98

Coconut Chai 99

Fat-Burning Vanilla Smoothie 100

Raspberry and Vanilla Smoothie 103

Creamy Orange Smoothie 104

Key Lime Smoothie 107

Almond Bliss Smoothie 108

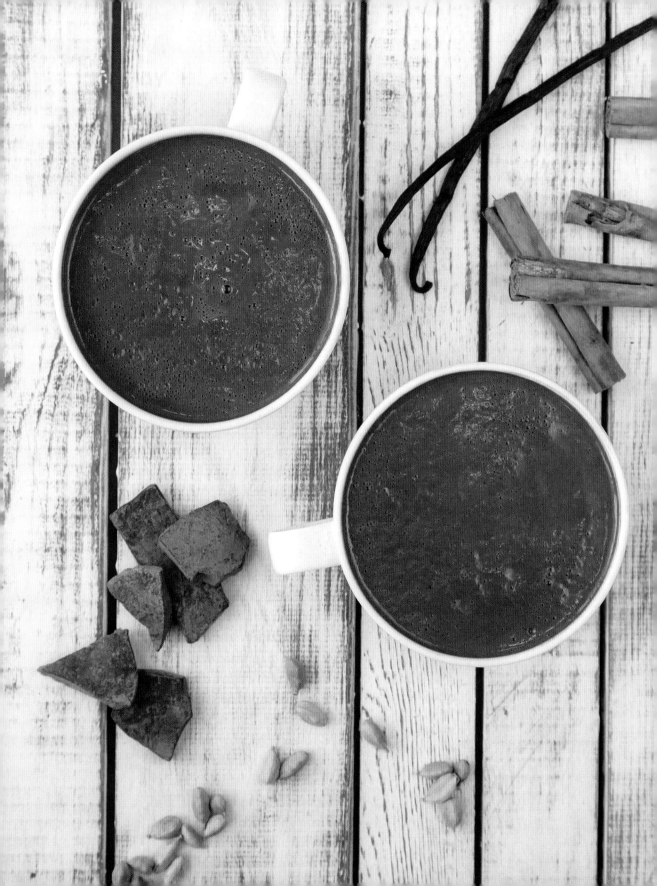

Creamy Dark Hot Chocolate

Made with pure dark chocolate, coconut milk, and spices, this is the Holy Grail for low-carb chocolate fiends. Treat yourself to a (guilt-free!) cup the next time a craving strikes. (Make this nut- and dairy-free by using coconut milk and water for the first two ingredients.)

½ cup (120 ml/4 fl oz) coconut milk or heavy whipping cream

½ cup (120 ml/4 fl oz) water or almond milk

2 cardamom pods, crushed

⅛ teaspoon ground cinnamon

¼ teaspoon sugar-free vanilla extract or ⅛ teaspoon vanilla powder

Pinch salt

2 tablespoons (20 g 0.7 ounce) granulated erythritol or Swerve

1 ounce (28 g) unsweetened chocolate

1 tablespoon (15 ml/0.5 fl oz) MCT oil or coconut oil

Few drops liquid stevia, to taste (optional)

—
Yield: 1 serving

In a small saucepan, combine the coconut milk, water, cardamom, cinnamon, vanilla, salt, and erythritol. Bring to a boil. When bubbles form on top, remove the mixture from the heat and let it sit for 5 minutes. Add the unsweetened chocolate and MCT oil and let it melt while stirring. If you want a sweeter taste, add the stevia and stir again.

Pour the chocolate mixture through a sieve into a blender and pulse for a few seconds until smooth and frothy. Serve hot!

NUTRITIONAL FACTS

Per serving: total carbs: 11.6 g; fiber: 4.2 g; net carbs: 7.4 g; protein: 6.3 g; fat: 52.9 g; energy: 528 kcal.

Macronutrient ratio: calories from carbs: 5 percent; protein: 5 percent; fat: 90 percent.

Creamy White Hot Chocolate

Never tried white hot chocolate? Now's the time! It's just as smooth and rich as its darker counterpart, and it's full of healthy fats—and it takes just five minutes to make.

½ cup (120 ml/4 fl oz) coconut milk or heavy whipping cream

½ cup (120 ml/4 fl oz) water or almond milk

¼ teaspoon sugar-free vanilla extract or ⅛ teaspoon vanilla powder

Pinch salt

1 tablespoon (10 g/0.4 oz) granulated erythritol or Swerve

1 ounce (28 g) Homemade White Chocolate (page 27)

1 tablespoon (15 ml/0.5 fl oz) MCT oil or coconut oil

Few drops liquid stevia, to taste (optional)

—
Yield: 1 serving

In a small saucepan, combine the coconut milk, water, vanilla, salt, and erythritol. Bring to a boil. When bubbles form on top, remove the mixture from the heat. Add the white chocolate and MCT oil and let it melt while stirring. If you want a sweeter taste, add the stevia and stir again. With a hand blender, pulse for a few seconds until smooth and frothy. Serve hot!

NUTRITIONAL FACTS

Per serving: total carbs: 6.5 g fiber: 0.1 g; net carbs: 6.4 g; protein: 3 g; fat: 57.8 g; energy: 536 kcal.

Macronutrient ratio: calories from carbs: 5 percent; protein: 2 percent; fat: 93 percent.

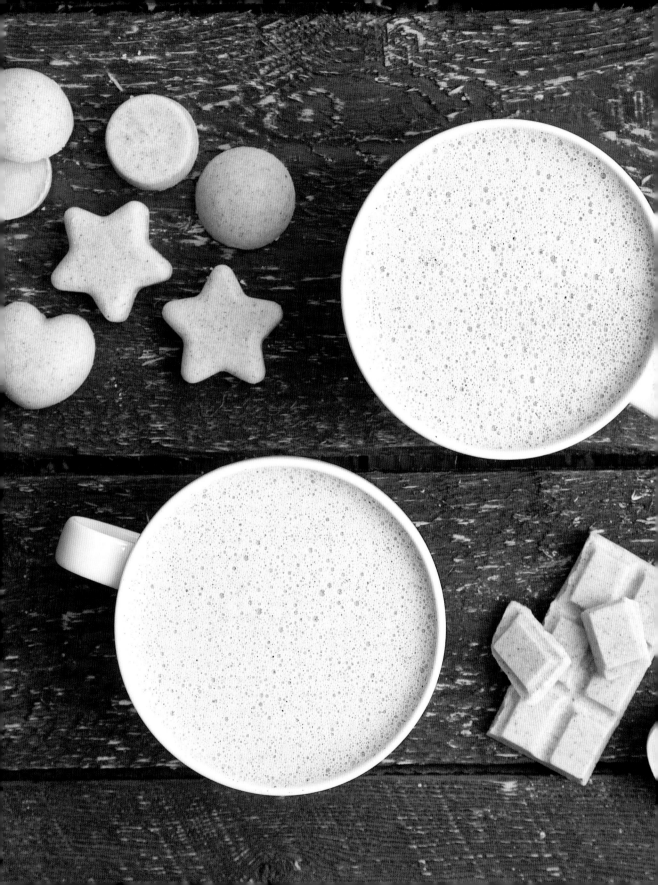

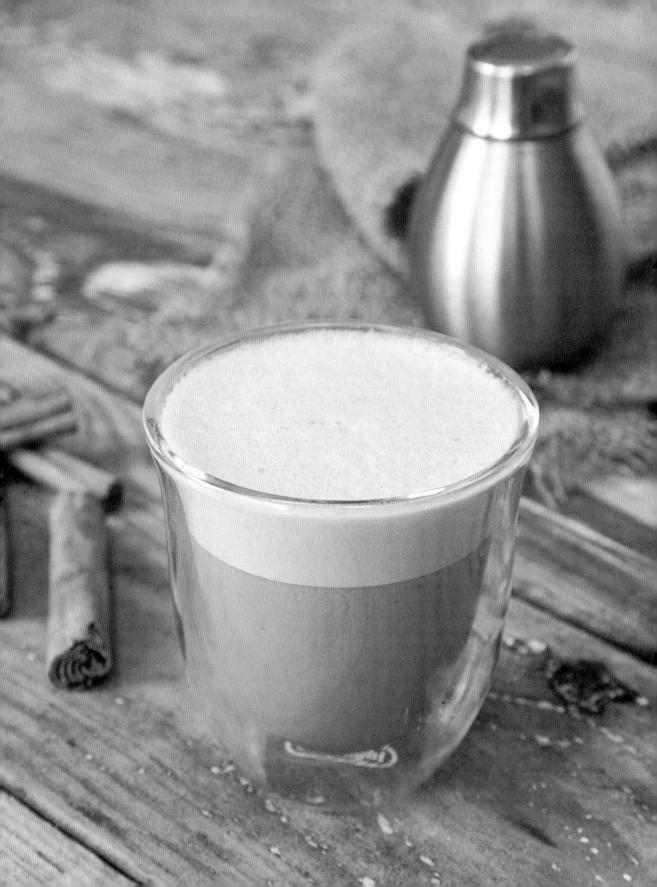

Creamy Keto Coffee

This is an upgraded version of the popular "bulletproof" coffee, which combines butter and coconut oil for a whack of healthy fats (and an instant energy boost). Here, egg yolks—don't worry, they won't scramble—add an amazingly creamy texture and make this recipe so filling and nutritious that it can replace a regular meal. (See also Coconut-Vanilla Coffee on page 98.)

1 cup (240 ml /8 fl oz) hot brewed coffee or black tea

1 tablespoon (15 ml/0.5 fl oz) coconut milk or heavy whipping cream

1 tablespoon (15 ml/0.5 fl oz) MCT oil or coconut oil

1 tablespoon (0.5 ounce, or 14 g) unsalted butter or more coconut oil

¼ to ½ teaspoon ground cinnamon or vanilla powder

3 large egg yolks, whites reserved for another use

1 tablespoon (10 g/0.4 oz) granulated erythritol or Swerve, or 3 to 5 drops liquid stevia (optional)

—
Yield: 1 serving

In a blender, combine the coffee, coconut milk, MCT oil, butter, cinnamon, and egg yolks. Pulse until smooth and frothy. If you want a sweeter taste, add the erythritol and pulse again. Serve hot!

NOTE:

Cutting down on caffeine? For a naturally caffeine-free alternative, try instant coffee powder made from chicory root or dandelion or make this recipe with your favorite caffeine-free tea instead.

NUTRITIONAL FACTS

Per serving: total carbs: 6.8 g; fiber: 0.4 g; net carbs: 6.4 g; protein: 8.8 g; fat: 42.3 g; energy: 436 kcal.

Macronutrient ratio: calories from carbs: 6 percent; protein: 8 percent; fat: 86 percent.

Coconut-Vanilla Coffee

In addition to Creamy Keto Coffee (page 97), here is another version of the popular "bulletproof coffee"—coffee with unsalted butter instead of cream—only without the butter, as MCT oil is more ketogenic.

1 cup (235 ml) hot brewed coffee

¼ cup (60 ml) unsweetened coconut milk

1 tablespoon (15 ml) MCT oil

18 drops liquid stevia (French vanilla flavor)

½ teaspoon vanilla extract

—
Yield: 1 serving

This is simple: Just combine everything in a blender and run until the coconut milk has melted and it's frothy.

NUTRITIONAL FACTS

Per serving: total carbs: 2 g; fiber: 0 g; net carbs: 2 g; protein: 1.1 g; fat: 22.4 g; calories: 215.

Macronutrient ratio: calories from carbs: 4 percent; protein: 2 percent; fat: 92 percent.

Cococcino

Here's a frosty, sweet coffee drink for all of you who have given up dairy—and it has no sugar. Think of the money you'll save! This is perfect on a hot summer day, or anytime.

1½ cups (355 ml) unsweetened coconut milk, chilled

⅔ cup (160 ml) brewed espresso, cooled

2 tablespoons (30 g) powdered Swerve

20 drops liquid stevia (vanilla, chocolate, hazelnut, or English toffee flavor)

About 10 ice cubes

—
Yield: 2 servings

Put everything but the ice in a blender and turn it on.

Drop in the ice cubes, one at a time, and run until the ice is pulverized. Pour and drink.

NUTRITIONAL FACTS

Per serving (13 oz, or 366 g): total carbs: 15 g; fiber: 0 g; net carbs: 15 g; protein: 2.4 g; fat: 25.1 g; calories: 280.

Macronutrient ratio: calories from carbs: 20 percent; protein: 3 percent; fat: 77 percent.

NOTE:

You can use sugar-free coffee-flavored syrup in place of the liquid stevia. It is less concentrated than liquid stevia; use to taste.

Coconut Chai

This spiced, sweetened Indian tea is commonly made with dairy milk, but coconut milk, also popular in India, works well here, too.

8 tea bags

4 cups (950 ml) water

½ teaspoon liquid stevia (plain or English toffee flavor)

1 teaspoon ground cinnamon

1 teaspoon ground cardamom

½ teaspoon ground nutmeg

½ teaspoon ground ginger

¼ teaspoon ground cloves

1¾ cups (410 ml) unsweetened coconut milk

—

Yield: 8 servings

In a big saucepan, combine everything but the coconut milk and bring to a boil. Turn off the burner and let it steep as it cools.

Strain through a fine-mesh strainer or let the spices settle to the bottom and pour off the tea as carefully as possible, leaving the powdery stuff behind.

Stir in the coconut milk. Store in the fridge and serve either hot or cold.

NUTRITIONAL FACTS

Per serving (6 oz, or 168 g):
total carbs: 1.4 g; fiber: 0 g;
net carbs: 1.4 g; protein: 0.7 g;
fat: 7.3 g; calories: 80.

Macronutrient ratio: calories from carbs: 7 percent; protein: 4 percent; fat: 89 percent.

NOTE:

Play around with the ingredients to your liking. For instance, sub in xylitol (2 heaping tablespoons [about 18 g]) for the stevia. Use heavy cream instead of the coconut milk—for 1 cup (235 ml) chai use ¼ cup (60 ml) cream. Optional: If using cream, make the tea ahead of time, keep it in the fridge, and then add the cream just before serving.

Fat-Burning Vanilla Smoothie

You don't need to get out the frying pan to have eggs for breakfast. It's so much faster to toss them into this thick, creamy smoothie! Combined with mascarpone cheese (or creamed coconut milk for a dairy-free version) and a dash of coconut oil, it's a full meal in a glass.

2 large egg yolks, whites reserved for another use

½ cup (120 g/4.2 oz) full-fat mascarpone cheese or creamed coconut milk

¼ cup (60 ml/2 fl oz) water

4 to 5 ice cubes

1 tablespoon (15 ml/0.5 fl oz) MCT oil or coconut oil (see Note)

1 teaspoon sugar-free vanilla extract or ½ teaspoon vanilla powder

1 tablespoon (10 g/0.4 oz) erythritol or Swerve, powdered, or 3 to 5 drops liquid stevia

Whipped cream or coconut milk, for topping (optional)

—

Yield: 1 serving

If using creamed coconut milk, make it a day ahead following the instructions on page 69. In a blender, combine the egg yolks, mascarpone, water, ice, MCT oil, vanilla, and erythritol. Pulse until smooth. Top with whipped cream or coconut milk (if using).

NOTE:

If you use coconut oil, it's important to make this using a blender to avoid leaving "pieces" of coconut oil in your smoothie. Unlike MCT oil, coconut oil is only liquid above 75°F (24°C). If you don't eat eggs, you can still enjoy this smoothie. Use 1 tablespoon (8 g/0.3 oz) of ground chia seeds or ¼ cup (25 g/0.9 oz) whey protein powder in place of the two egg yolks.

NUTRITIONAL FACTS

Per serving: total carbs: 4.6 g; fiber: 0.9 g; net carbs: 3.7 g; protein: 12.2 g; fat: 64.3 g; energy: 649 kcal.

Macronutrient ratio: calories from carbs: 2 percent; protein: 8 percent; fat: 90 percent.

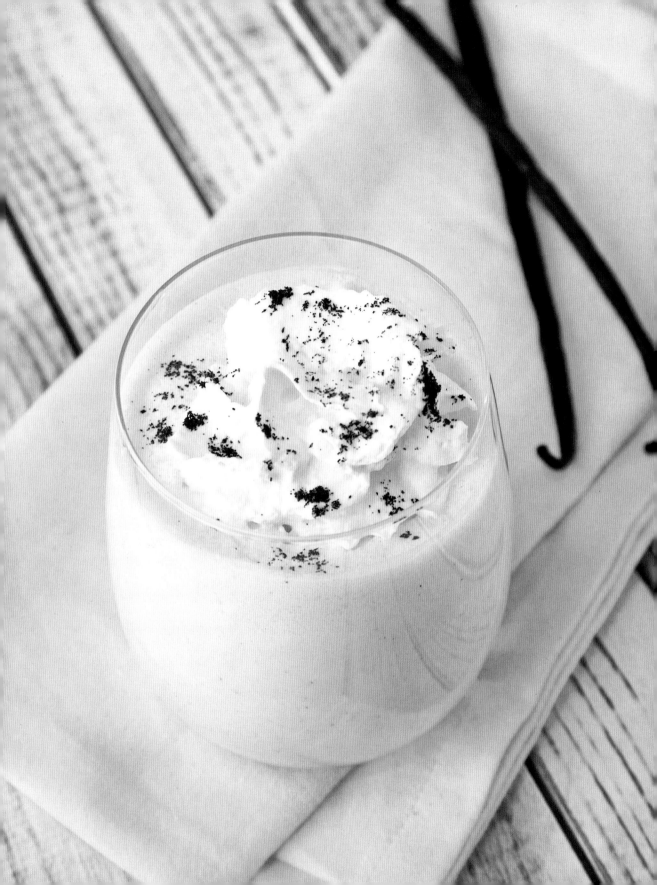

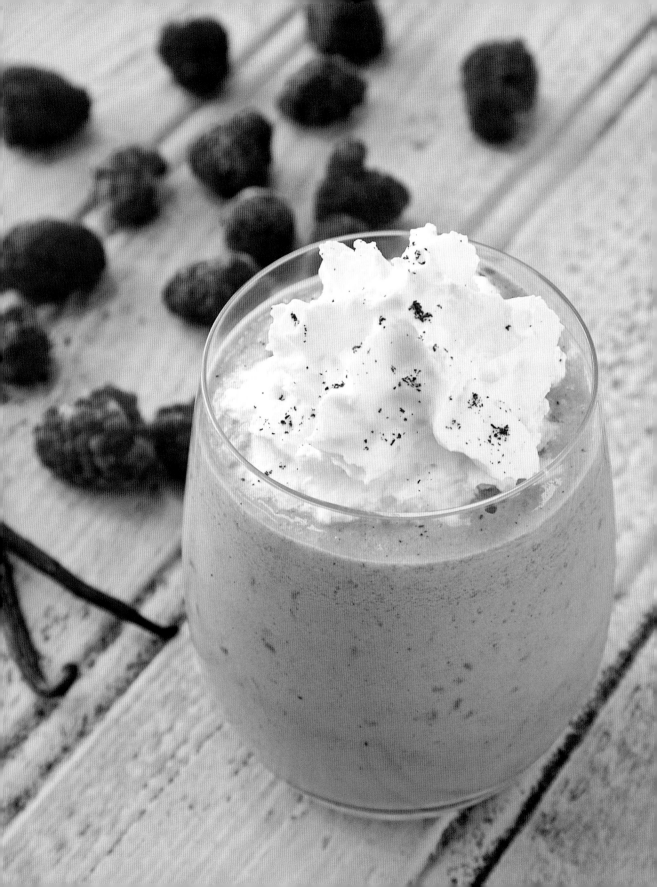

Raspberry and Vanilla Smoothie

This liquid fat bomb is another great breakfast option. It's loaded with raspberries, mascarpone, and good-for-you fats, and it's perfect for summer mornings when the weather's too warm for a hot meal.

⅓ cup (50 g/1.8 oz) raspberries, fresh or frozen

½ cup (120 g/4.2 oz) mascarpone cheese or creamed coconut milk (see page 69)

¼ cup (60 ml/2 fl oz) water

4 to 5 ice cubes

½ teaspoon sugar-free vanilla extract or ¼ teaspoon vanilla powder

1 tablespoon (15 ml/0.5 fl oz) MCT oil or coconut oil (see Note)

1 tablespoon (10 g/0.4 oz) erythritol or Swerve, powdered, or 3 to 5 drops liquid stevia (optional)

Whipped cream or coconut milk, for topping (optional)

—
Yield: 1 serving

If using creamed coconut milk, make it a day ahead following the instructions on page 69.

In a blender, combine the raspberries, mascarpone, water, ice, vanilla, and MCT oil. Pulse until smooth. If you want a sweeter taste, add the erythritol and top with whipped cream.

> **NOTE:**
>
> If you use coconut oil, it's important to make this using a blender to avoid leaving "pieces" of coconut oil in your smoothie. Unlike MCT oil, coconut oil is only liquid above 75°F (24°C).

NUTRITIONAL FACTS

Per serving: total carbs: 5.8 g; fiber: 1.3 g; net carbs: 4.6 g; protein: 7.5 g; fat: 55.5 g; energy: 552 kcal.

Macronutrient ratio: calories from carbs: 3 percent; protein: 6 percent; fat: 91 percent.

Creamy Orange Smoothie

Creamy and tangy all at once, this citrusy smoothie is as refreshing as the ice pops we loved as kids—but it's far more nutritious and filling, and, of course, it's completely sugar free.

2 large egg yolks, whites reserved for another use

½ cup (120 g/4.2 oz) full-fat mascarpone cheese or creamed coconut milk

¼ cup (60 ml/2 fl oz) water

4 to 5 ice cubes

1 tablespoon (15 ml/0.5 fl oz) MCT oil or coconut oil (see Note)

1 teaspoon freshly grated orange zest or ¼ to ½ teaspoon sugar-free orange extract

¼ teaspoon ground cinnamon

1 tablespoon (10 g/0.4 oz) erythritol or Swerve, powdered, or 3 to 5 drops liquid stevia

Whipped cream or coconut milk, for topping (optional)

—
Yield: 1 serving

If using creamed coconut milk, make it a day ahead following the instructions on page 69.

In a blender, combine the egg yolks, mascarpone, water, ice, MCT oil, orange zest, cinnamon, and erythritol. Pulse until smooth. Top with whipped cream (if using) and serve.

NOTE:

If you use coconut oil, it's important to make this using a blender to avoid leaving "pieces" of coconut oil in your smoothie. Unlike MCT oil, coconut oil is only liquid above 75°F (24°C). If you don't eat eggs, you can still enjoy this smoothie. Use 1 tablespoon (8 g/0.3 oz) of ground chia seeds or ¼ cup (25 g/0.9 oz) whey protein powder in place of the two egg yolks.

NUTRITIONAL FACTS

Per serving: total carbs: 4.9 g; fiber: 0.6 g; net carbs: 4.3 g; protein: 12.3 g; fat: 64.4 g; energy: 648 kcal.

Macronutrient ratio: calories from carbs: 3 percent; protein: 7 percent; fat: 90 percent.

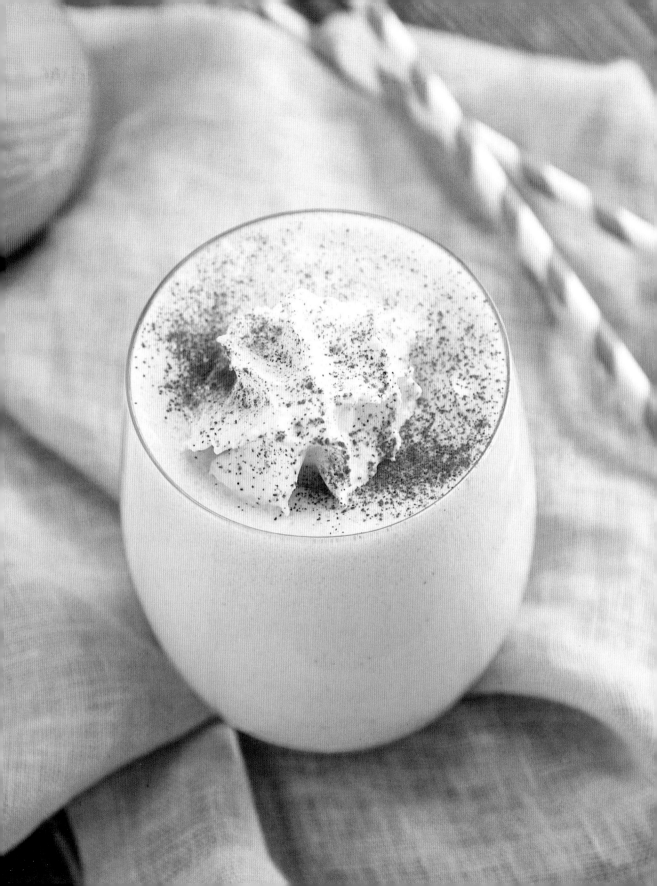

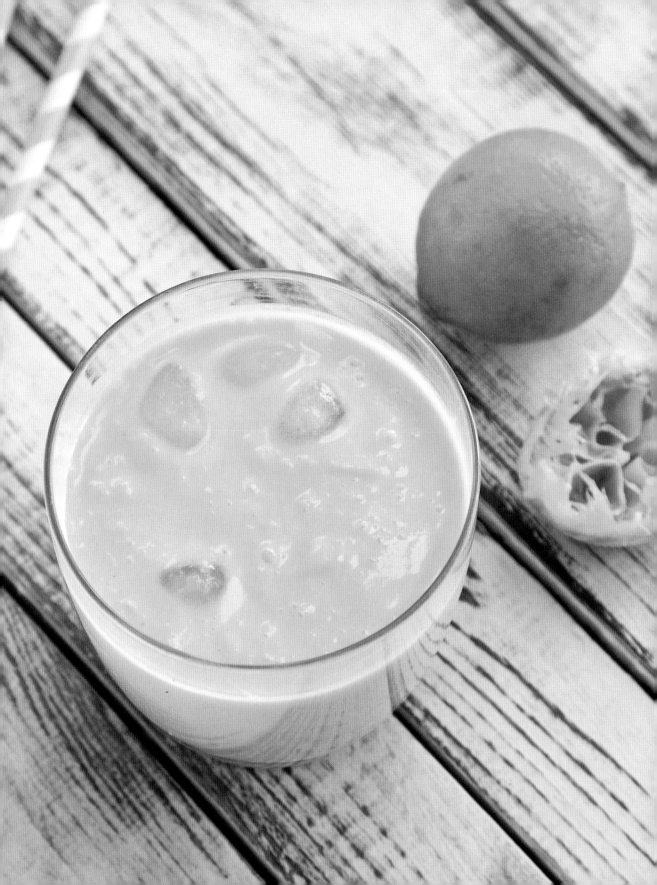

Key Lime Smoothie

Never had avocado for breakfast before? Well, there's a first time for everything! Avocados are so nutritious, plus they're a great flavor match for lime and they add a velvety texture to this satisfying, low-carb smoothie.

½ medium (75 g/2.6 oz) ripe avocado, pitted and peeled

¼ cup (60 ml/2 fl oz) creamed coconut milk or heavy whipping cream

½ cup (120 ml/4 fl oz) water

4 to 5 ice cubes

1 tablespoon (15 ml/0.5 fl oz) MCT oil or coconut oil (see Note)

2 tablespoons (30 ml/1 fl oz) freshly squeezed lime juice

1 teaspoon freshly grated lime zest

1 tablespoon (10 g/0.4 oz) erythritol or Swerve, powdered, or 3 to 5 drops liquid stevia

Whipped cream or coconut milk, for topping (optional)

—
Yield: 1 serving

If using creamed coconut milk, make it a day ahead following the instructions on page 69. In a blender, combine the avocado, creamed coconut milk, water, ice, MCT oil, lime juice, lime zest, and erythritol. Pulse until smooth. Top with whipped cream (if using), and serve.

NOTE:

If you use coconut oil, it's important to make this using a blender to avoid leaving "pieces" of coconut oil in your smoothie. Unlike MCT oil, coconut oil is only liquid above 75°F (24°C).

NUTRITIONAL FACTS

Per serving: total carbs: 10.1 g; fiber: 5.3 g net carbs: 4.8 g; protein: 5 g; fat: 45.2 g; energy: 454 kcal.

Macronutrient ratio: calories from carbs: 4 percent; protein: 5 percent; fat: 91 percent.

Almond Bliss Smoothie

Chocolate, coconut, and almond—three ingredients usually found in your favorite candy bar. Transform them into a healthy smoothie with this sippable fat bomb recipe.

½ cup (120 ml/4 fl oz) coconut milk or heavy whipping cream

½ cup (120 ml/4 fl oz) almond milk

1 tablespoon (8 g/0.3 oz) chia seeds

2 tablespoons (32 g/1.1 oz) Almond Bliss Butter (page 22)

1 tablespoon (15 ml/0.5 fl oz) MCT oil or coconut oil (see Note)

1 tablespoon (10 g/0.4 oz) erythritol or Swerve, powdered, or 3 to 5 drops liquid stevia

1 teaspoon toasted, unsweetened shredded coconut or whipped cream, for topping (optional)

—
Yield: 1 serving

In a blender, combine the coconut milk, almond milk, and chia seeds. Let the mixture soak for 5 to 10 minutes. Add the Almond Bliss Butter, MCT oil, and erythritol. Pulse until smooth and creamy. Top with toasted coconut or whipped cream (if using), and serve.

NOTE

If you use coconut oil, it's important to make this using a blender to avoid leaving "pieces" of coconut oil in your smoothie. Unlike MCT oil, coconut oil is only liquid above 75°F (24°C).

NUTRITIONAL FACTS

Per serving: total carbs: 13.6 g; fiber: 6.3 g; net carbs: 7.3 g; protein: 8.8 g; fat: 53.7 g; energy: 548 kcal.

Macronutrient ratio: calories from carbs: 5 percent; protein: 6 percent; fat: 89 percent.

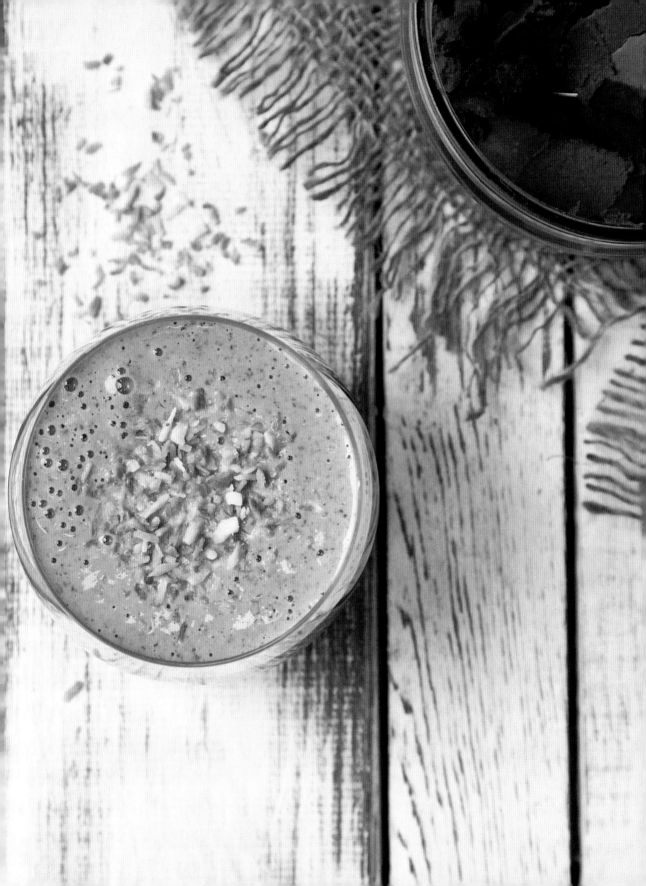

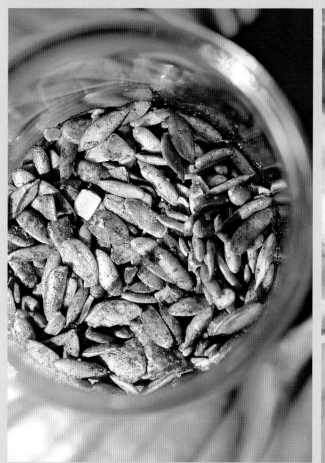

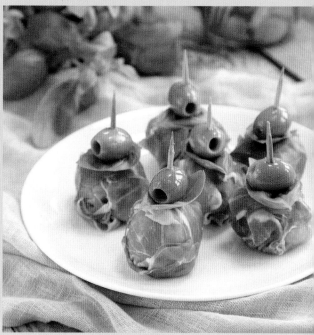

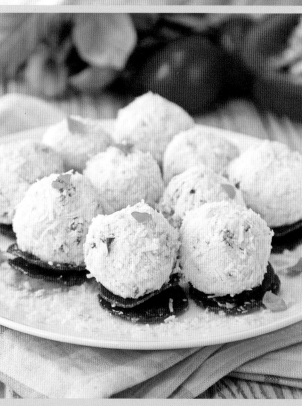

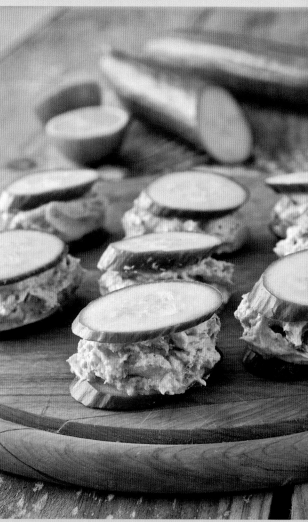

6

SAFE SNACKING: Nut-Free, Dairy-Free, and Egg-Free Options

Welcome to an entirely nut-free chapter! Although there are nut-free recipes throughout the book, we've gathered twenty in one chapter for easy selection. Some of these recipes are also dairy-free (Sweet Bacon Kale) or egg-free (Pepperoni Pizza Fat Bombs).

Whether a food allergy affects you directly, it's likely you will face a time when you need to prepare a snack for yourself or someone who is affected, such as family, friends, or coworkers. Globally, an estimated 220 million people have food allergies, including 15 million Americans, according to End Allergies Together.

With these statistics in mind, we've made it easy so you can prepare your own safe snacks with worry-free confidence. What's more, excluding certain allergy-related foods doesn't mean you have to skimp on protein, healthy fats, or flavor. Enjoy these delicious sweet and savory snacks!

Sweet & Salty Spiced Pepitas 113

Crispy Okra Sticks 113

Pepperoni Pizza Fat Bombs 114

Stilton and Chive Fat Bombs 117

Bacon and Guacamole Fat Bombs 118

Ham and Cheese Fat Bombs 121

Veggie and Cheese Fat Bombs 122

Smoked Mackerel Pâté Fat Bombs 125

Earl Grey Truffles 126

Toasted Coconut Cups 128

Chewy Hempseed Squares 130

Chocolate-Avocado Truffles 132

Chocolate Chia Workout Bars 135

Cinnamon Donut Holes 136

Sweet Bacon Kale 138

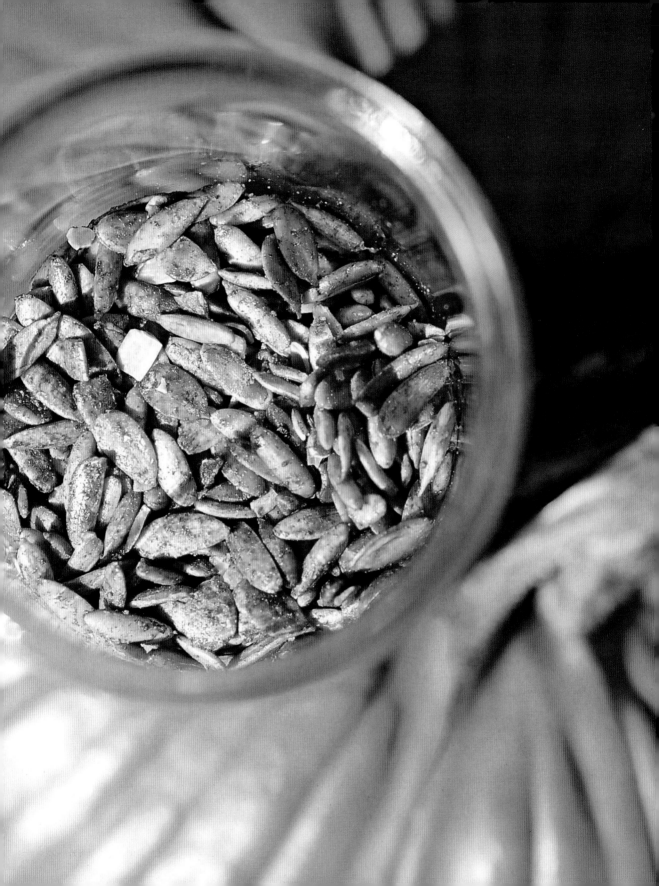

Sweet & Salty Spiced Pepitas

Pepitas are a wonderful snack because they are high in both iron and zinc, which are vital for enhancing memory, and great for strengthening your immune system and helping boost energy. Moreover, they have a perfect crunch. Add a little salt and a little sweetness and you have a fabulously addictive snack!

2 cups (450 g) raw pepitas

2 teaspoons pumpkin pie spice

1 teaspoon salt

1½ tablespoons (30 g) maple syrup

—

Yield: 2 cups (450 g)

Preheat the oven to 350°F (180°C, or gas mark 4). Line a baking sheet with parchment paper.

In a medium bowl, mix together the pepitas, pumpkin pie spice, and salt. Add the maple syrup and stir until the pumpkin seed mixture is evenly coated. Spread out the seeds evenly on the prepared baking sheet and bake for 12 minutes, or until they start to turn brown, stirring halfway through so they bake evenly. Take out of the oven and allow to cool for at least 30 minutes. As they cool, they will get even crunchier! Store in an airtight container.

NUTRITIONAL FACTS

Per ¼-cup serving (11/3 oz, or 37 g): total carbs: 6.3 g; fiber: 2 g; net carbs: 4.3 g; protein: 9.8 g; fat: 15.9 g; calories: 191.

Macronutrient ratio: calories from carbs: 12 percent; protein: 19 percent; fat: 69 percent.

Crispy Okra Sticks

These are a good go-to snack whenever you're in the mood for something crispy and salty. Eat them while they are fresh out of the oven and they will make traditional potato chips seem boring and bland.

½ pound (225 g) fresh okra

1 to 2 tablespoons (13.5 to 27 g) coconut oil, melted

¼ teaspoon salt

—

Yield: about 4 servings

Preheat the oven to 425°F (220°C, or gas mark 7). Rinse and dry the okra and then slice each pod in half lengthwise. Place in a mixing bowl and coat in melted coconut oil and salt. Lay the okra flat on a baking sheet (without parchment paper) and bake for 10 minutes. Turn the okra and bake for another 10 minutes, or until crispy. Serve immediately.

NUTRITIONAL FACTS

Per serving (2 oz, or 60 g): total carbs: 4.2 g; fiber: 1.8 g; net carbs: 2.4 g; protein: 1.1 g; fat: 3.5 g; calories: 49.

Macronutrient ratio: calories from carbs: 32 percent; protein: 8 percent; fat: 60 percent.

Pepperoni Pizza Fat Bombs

These keto-friendly fat bombs are every bit as good as delivery pepperoni pizza—minus the carb-laden crust, of course!

3.5 ounces (100 g) full-fat cream cheese, at room temperature

¼ cup (56 g/2 oz) unsalted butter, at room temperature

12 (36 g/1.3 oz) pepperoni slices

1 clove of garlic, minced

½ small red pepper (40 g/1.4 oz), finely chopped

¼ cup (28 g/1 oz) grated mozzarella cheese

1 to 2 tablespoons (5 to 10 g/ 0.2 to 0.4 oz) chopped fresh herbs (such as basil, oregano, thyme), or 1 to 2 teaspoons dried herbs

⅛ teaspoon chili powder

Pinch salt

½ cup (30 g/1.1 oz) grated Parmesan cheese

—
Yield: 6 servings

NUTRITIONAL FACTS

Per serving: total carbs: 1.5 g; fiber: 0.2 g; net carbs: 1.3 g; protein: 5.7 g; fat: 17.2 g; energy: 175 kcal.

Macronutrient ratio: calories from carbs: 3 percent; protein: 12 percent; fat: 85 percent.

In a bowl, mash together the cream cheese and the butter with a fork, or process in a food processor until smooth.

In a large skillet set over medium heat, cook the pepperoni slices and on both sides until crispy. Transfer to a plate to cool.

Add the garlic and red pepper to the pepperoni juices in the skillet and cook for a few minutes over medium heat until fragrant. Remove from the heat and cool slightly. Add to the cream cheese and butter mixture and mix well with an electric beater or a hand whisk.

Add the grated mozzarella cheese, herbs, chili powder, and salt. Mix well again. Refrigerate for 20 to 30 minutes, or until set.

Using a large spoon or an ice cream scoop, divide the mixture into six balls. Roll each ball in the Parmesan cheese and place on top of two slices of crisped pepperoni. Enjoy immediately or refrigerate in an airtight container for up to 5 days.

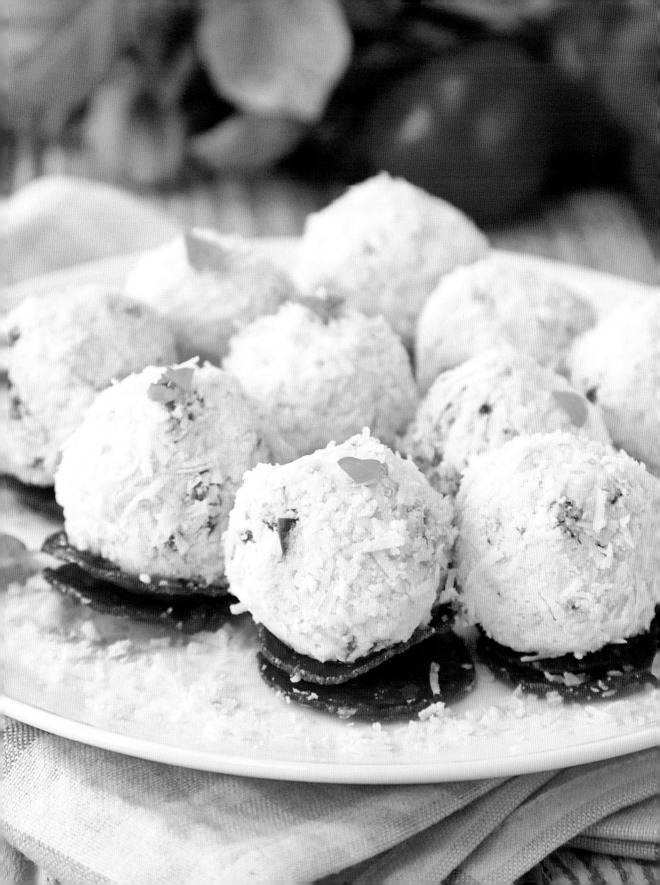

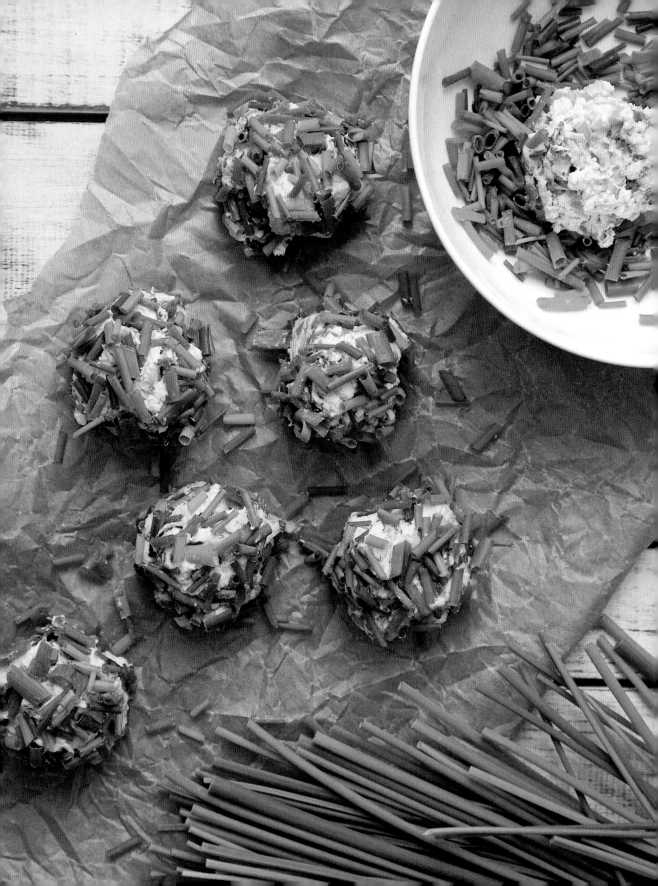

Stilton and Chive Fat Bombs

Blue cheese addicts will adore these zero-carb fat bombs, in which pungent Stilton is suspended in a cloud of cream cheese and butter. The final flourish comes from a thorough coating of freshly chopped chives.

3.5 ounces (100 g) full-fat cream cheese, at room temperature

¼ cup (56 g/2 oz) unsalted butter, at room temperature

½ cup (65 g/2.3 oz) crumbled Stilton or other blue cheese

2 medium (30 g/1.1 oz) spring onions, finely chopped

1 tablespoon (3 g/0.1 oz) finely chopped fresh parsley

Pinch salt

⅓ cup (30 g/1.1 oz) chopped fresh chives, or more finely chopped spring onion

—

Yield: 6 servings

In a bowl, mash together the cream cheese and butter, or process in a food processor until smooth.

Add the crumbled Stilton, spring onions, and parsley. Mix until well combined. Season with salt. Refrigerate for 20 to 30 minutes, or until set.

Using a large spoon or an ice cream scoop, divide the mixture into six balls. Roll each ball in the chopped chives and place on a plate. Enjoy immediately or refrigerate in an airtight container for up to 5 days.

NUTRITIONAL FACTS

Per serving: total carbs: 1.1 g; fiber: 0.2 g; net carbs: 0.8 g; protein: 4.5 g; fat: 16.2 g; energy: 157 kcal.

Macronutrient ratio: calories from carbs: 2 percent; protein: 11 percent; fat: 87 percent.

Bacon and Guacamole Fat Bombs

There's only one way to improve upon homemade guacamole, and that's to transform it into bacon-coated fat bombs. Seriously.

4 large bacon slices
(120 g/4.2 oz)

½ large (100 g /3.5 oz) avocado, halved, pitted, and peeled

¼ cup (56 g /2 oz) unsalted butter or ghee, at room temperature

2 garlic cloves, crushed

1 small chile pepper, finely chopped

1 tablespoon (15 ml/0.5 fl oz) fresh lime juice

Salt and pepper, to taste

½ small (35 g /1.2 oz) white onion, diced

—
Yield: 6 servings

NUTRITIONAL FACTS

Per serving: total carbs: 2.7 g; fiber: 1.3 g; net carbs: 1.4 g; protein: 3.4 g; fat: 15.2 g; energy: 156 kcal.

Macronutrient ratio: calories from carbs: 3 percent; protein: 9 percent; fat: 88 percent.

Preheat the oven to 375°F (/190°C, or gas mark 5). Line a rimmed baking sheet with parchment paper. Be sure to use a rimmed sheet to contain the bacon fat, as you'll need it for the recipe, too. Lay the bacon strips flat on the parchment, leaving enough space between so they don't overlap. Place the sheet in the preheated oven and cook for 10 to 15 minutes, or until crispy. The exact amount of cooking time depends on the thickness of the bacon slices. Remove from the oven and set aside to cool. When cool enough to handle, crumble the bacon into a bowl and set aside.

In a bowl, combine the avocado, butter, garlic, chile pepper, and lime juice. Season with salt and pepper. Mash with a potato masher or fork until well combined. Stir in the onion. Pour in the bacon grease from the baking sheet and mix well. Cover with aluminum foil and refrigerate for 20 to 30 minutes.

Using a large spoon or an ice cream scoop, divide the mixture into 6 balls. If serving immediately, roll them in the crumbled bacon. If serving later, refrigerate without the bacon coating in an airtight container for up to 5 days. Roll the fat bombs in freshly cooked or reheated bacon crumbs just before serving.

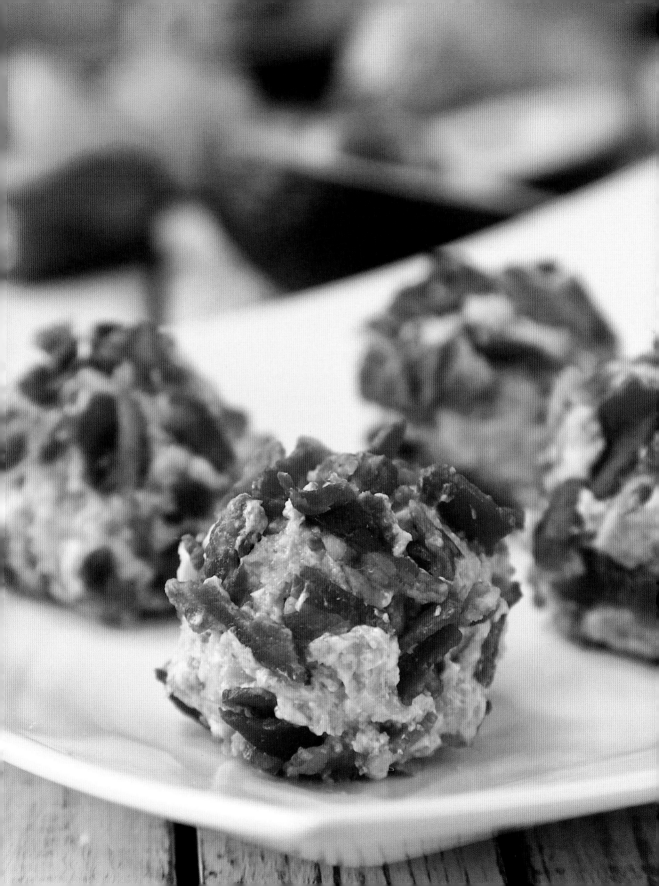

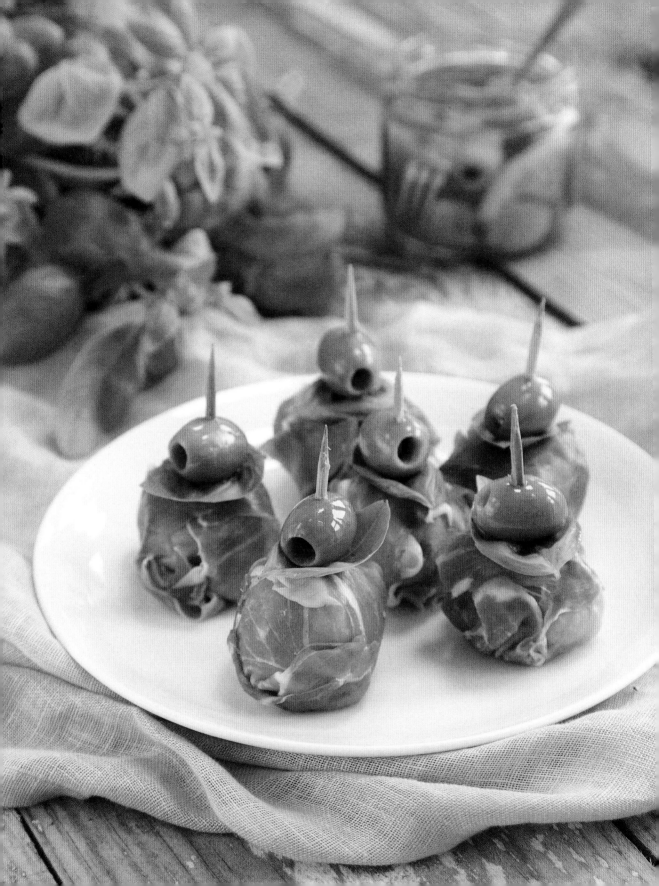

Ham and Cheese Fat Bombs

There are few things that can't be improved by a cloak of sweet-and-salty Parma ham—and these creamy, basil-flecked fat bombs are no exception. Try them as a low-carb afternoon snack.

3.5 ounces (100 g) full-fat cream cheese, at room temperature

¼ cup (56 g/2 oz) unsalted butter, at room temperature

¼ cup (30 g/1.1 oz) grated Cheddar or Gouda cheese

2 tablespoons (10 g/0.4 oz) chopped fresh basil

Salt and pepper, to taste

6 slices (90 g/3.2 oz) Parma ham

6 large (30 g/1.1 oz) green olives, pitted

—
Yield: 6 servings

In a bowl, mash together the cream cheese and butter, or process in a food processor until smooth.

Add the Cheddar and basil and mix until well combined. Season with salt and pepper. Refrigerate for 20 to 30 minutes, or until set.

Using a large spoon or an ice-cream scoop, divide the mixture into six balls. Wrap each ball in one slice of Parma ham and place on a plate. Top each ball with one olive and pierce with a toothpick to hold it in place. Enjoy immediately or refrigerate in an airtight container for up to 5 days.

NUTRITIONAL FACTS

Per serving: total carbs: 0.9 g; fiber: 0.2 g; net carbs: 0.7 g; protein: 6.4 g; fat: 16.4 g; energy: 167 kcal.

Macronutrient ratio: calories from carbs: 2 percent; protein: 14 percent; fat: 84 percent.

Veggie and Cheese Fat Bombs

Just like a gourmet vegetable pizza only *sans* carbs, these tasty fat bombs feature caramelized onion, porcini mushrooms, fresh spinach, and goat cheese.

3.5 ounces (100 g) full-fat cream cheese, at room temperature

¼ cup (56 g/2 oz) unsalted butter, at room temperature

1 tablespoon (15 g/0.5 oz) ghee

½ small (35 g/1.2 oz) white onion, peeled and finely chopped

1 clove of garlic, peeled and finely chopped

½ cup (15 g/0.5 oz) dried porcini mushrooms, soaked in 1 cup (235 ml) warm water for 30 minutes and then drained and sliced

2 cups (60 g/2.1 oz) fresh spinach

Salt and pepper, to taste

¼ cup (30 g/2.1 oz) grated hard goat cheese

—
Yield: 6 servings

In a bowl, mash together the cream cheese and butter, or process in a food processor until smooth.

Grease a hot pan with the ghee. Add the onion and garlic and cook over medium heat for 2 to 3 minutes, or until fragrant. Add the mushrooms and cook for about 2 minutes more. Add the spinach and cook for 1 minute more, or until wilted. Remove the pan from the heat and set aside to cool.

Add the cooled mushroom and spinach mixture to the cream cheese and butter and mix until well combined. Season with salt and pepper. Refrigerate for 20 to 30 minutes, or until set.

Using a large spoon or an ice cream scoop, divide the mixture into six balls. Roll each ball in the goat cheese. Enjoy immediately or refrigerate in an airtight container for up to 5 days.

NUTRITIONAL FACTS

Per serving: total carbs: 3.6 g; fiber: 0.6 g; net carbs: 3 g; protein: 3.4 g; fat: 16.7 g; energy: 166 kcal.

Macronutrient ratio: calories from carbs: 7 percent; protein: 8 percent; fat: 85 percent.

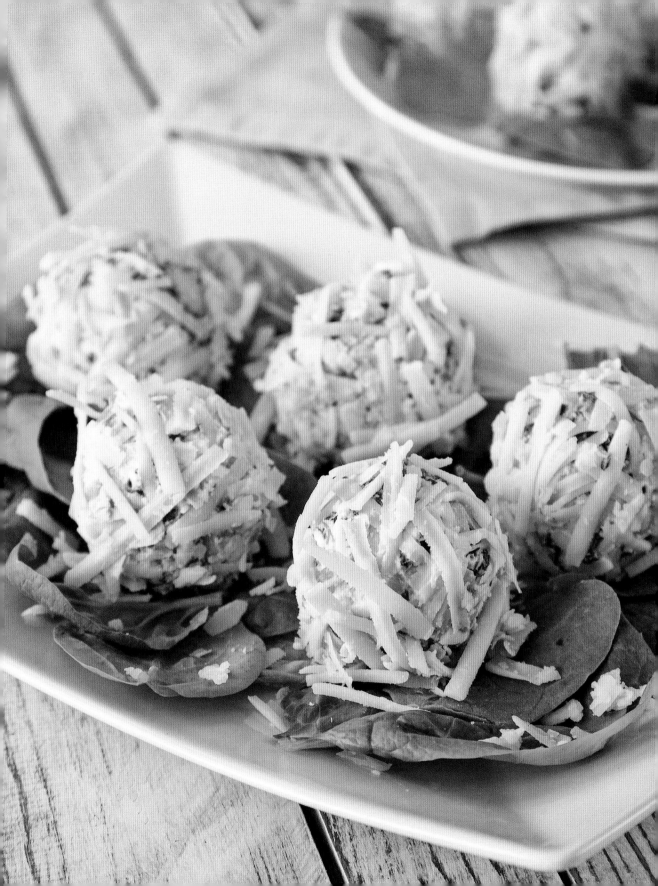

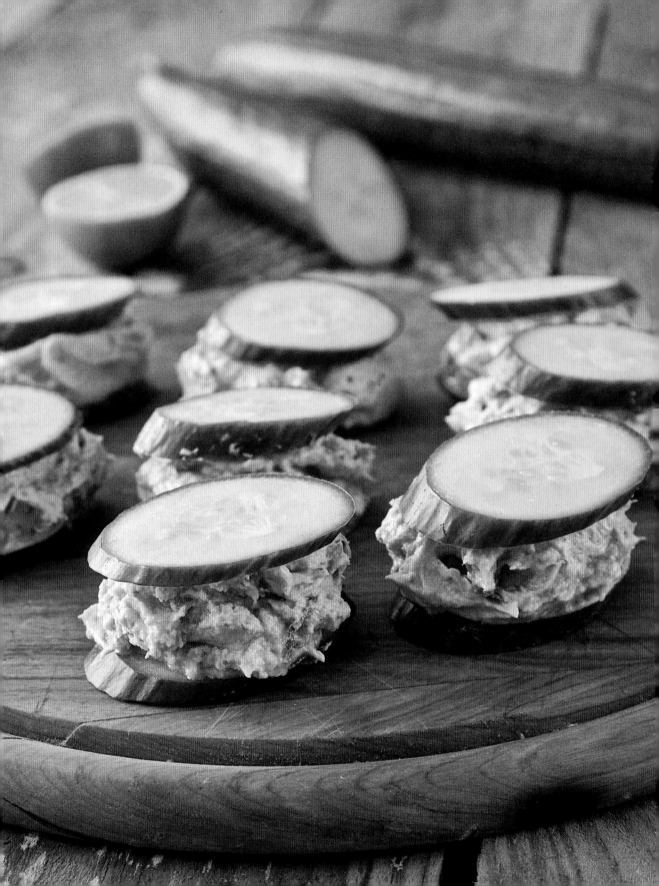

Smoked Mackerel Pâté Fat Bombs

If you're a fan of smoked fish, you're sure to love this low-carb dip. It's lightened and brightened by a dash of fresh lime juice and a handful of chives.

3.5 ounces (100 g) full-fat cream cheese, at room temperature

¼ cup (56 g/2 oz) unsalted butter, at room temperature

1 medium (100 g/3.5 oz) smoked mackerel fillet

1 tablespoon (15 ml/0.5 fl oz) freshly squeezed lime juice

2 tablespoons (8 g/0.3 oz) chopped fresh chives

Cucumber slices, for serving (optional)

—
Yield: 6 servings

In a food processor, combine the cream cheese, butter, mackerel, and lime juice. Pulse until smooth. Transfer to a bowl, add the chives, and mix with a spoon. Refrigerate for 20 to 30 minutes, or until set. Enjoy as a dip with cucumber slices, or refrigerate in an airtight container for up to 1 week.

NUTRITIONAL FACTS

Per serving: total carbs: 0.8 g; fiber: 0.1 g; net carbs: 0.7 g; protein: 4.9 g; fat: 16.5 g; energy: 161 kcal.

Macronutrient ratio: calories from carbs: 2 percent; protein: 11 percent; fat: 87 percent.

Earl Grey Truffles

Earl Grey tea adds a haunting, delicate flavor to these dark chocolate truffles. Be sure to use high-quality tea: it really does yield a better result.

FOR TRUFFLES:

⅔ cup (150 ml /5 fl oz) coconut milk or heavy whipping cream

½ cup (80 g/2.8 oz) powdered erythritol or Swerve

¼ cup (2 ounces, or 56 g) unsalted butter, ghee, or coconut oil, at room temperature

1 tablespoon (5 g/0.2 oz) good-quality earl grey tea leaves

6 ounces (170 g) unsweetened chocolate, broken into small pieces

Pinch salt

Few drops liquid stevia, to taste (optional)

1 tablespoon (14 g/0.5 oz) macadamia oil or other light-tasting oil, for shaping the truffles

FOR COATING:

4.2 ounces (120 g) Homemade White Chocolate (page 27)

2 tablespoons (28 g/1 oz) cacao nibs

—

Yield: 14 servings

NUTRITIONAL FACTS

Per serving (1 truffle): total carbs: 5.1 g; fiber: 2 g; net carbs: 3.1 g; protein: 2.5 g; fat: 20.1 g; energy: 208 kcal.

Macronutrient ratio: calories from carbs: 6 percent; protein: 5 percent; fat: 89 percent.

TO MAKE THE TRUFFLES: In a saucepan, combine the coconut milk, erythritol, and butter. Bring to a boil. Immediately remove the mixture from the heat and stir in the tea. Cover and let sit for 5 to 10 minutes.

In a bowl, place the unsweetened chocolate piece. Through a sieve, slowly pour the hot coconut milk over the chocolate, pressing on the tea leaves as the sieve catches them. Discard the tea leaves. Stir until the chocolate is completely melted and smooth. If the chocolate mixture separates, add a splash of boiling water or place in a blender and process until smooth. Add the salt. If you want a sweeter taste, add the stevia. Cool and refrigerate for 1 hour, or until firm.

To shape the truffles, dip a spoon or melon baller in warm water and scoop out fourteen balls of the chilled mixture. Lightly coat your hands in macadamia oil. Roll the truffles between your palms to form spheres about twice the size of "standard" truffles. Place on a parchment-lined tray and freeze for about 30 minutes.

TO MAKE THE COATING: Melt the white chocolate in a double boiler, or heat-proof bowl placed over a small saucepan filled with 1 cup of water, over medium heat. Once melted, remove from the heat and set aside to cool.

Gently pierce each frozen truffle with a toothpick or a fork. Working one at a time, hold each truffle over the melted white chocolate and spoon the chocolate over it to coat completely. Turn the stick as you work until the coating is solidified. Place the coated truffles on a parchment-lined tray and drizzle any remaining coating over them. Before the truffles become completely solid, sprinkle them with the cacao nibs.

Refrigerate the coated truffles for at least 15 minutes to harden. Keep refrigerated for up to 1 week or freeze for up to 3 months.

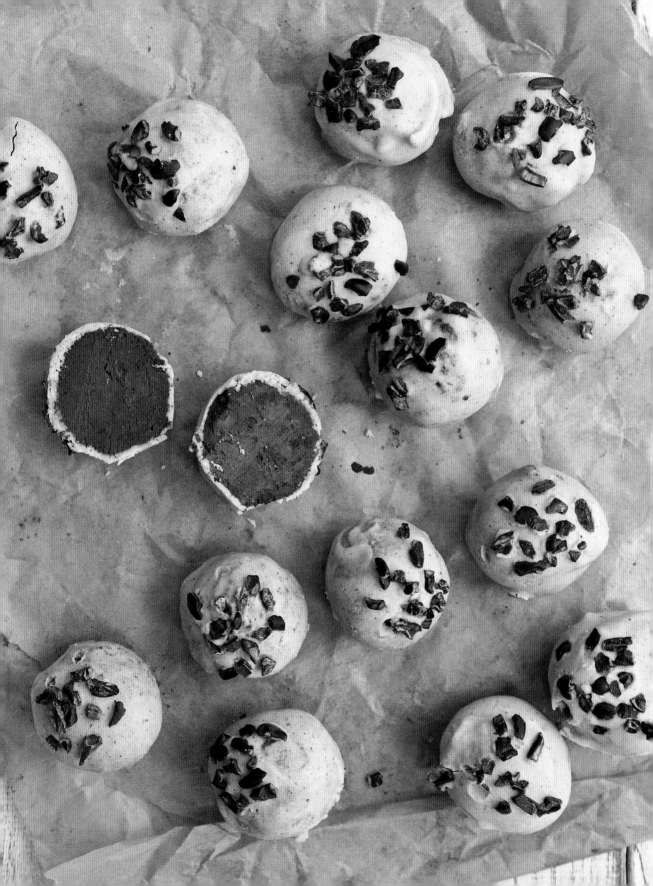

Toasted Coconut Cups

These cups are surprisingly easy to make! Toasting the coconut brings out its natural sweetness and adds some crunch.

1½ cups (112 g/4 oz) unsweetened desiccated, shredded, or flaked coconut

¼ cup (55 g/1.9 oz) extra virgin coconut oil, at room temperature

¼ cup (56 g/2 oz) unsalted butter, or more coconut oil, at room temperature

¼ teaspoon ground cinnamon or vanilla powder

Pinch salt

Few drops liquid stevia, to taste, or 2 tablespoons (0.7 ounce, or 20 g) erythritol or Swerve, powdered (optional)

—
Yield: 12 servings

NUTRITIONAL FACTS

Per serving (1 fat bomb): total carbs: 2.6 g; fiber: 1.9 g; net carbs: 0.7 g; protein: 1.9 g; fat: 9.6 g; energy: 104 kcal.

Macronutrient ratio: calories from carbs: 3 percent; protein: 8 percent; fat: 89 percent.

Preheat the oven to 350°F (175°C, or gas mark 4). Spread the coconut on a baking sheet. Place it in the oven and toast for 5 to 8 minutes, or until lightly golden. Stir once or twice to prevent burning. Remove from the oven and cool for 5 minutes. Transfer to a food processor and pulse until smooth. This may take time. At first, the mixture will be dry. Scrape down the sides of your processor several times with a rubber spatula if the mixture sticks. The final consistency should be smooth and runny.

Add the coconut oil. Then add the butter, 2 tablespoons (28 g) at a time, pulsing after each addition. Add the cinnamon and salt. Pulse to mix well. If you want a sweeter taste, add the stevia and pulse again.

Fill a mini muffin tin or ice cube tray with 2 tablespoon (20g/ 0.7 oz) portions. It should yield twelve servings. Refrigerate for at least 30 minutes, or until solid. Keep refrigerated for up to 1 week, as the coconut oil and butter become very soft at room temperature, or freeze for up to 3 months.

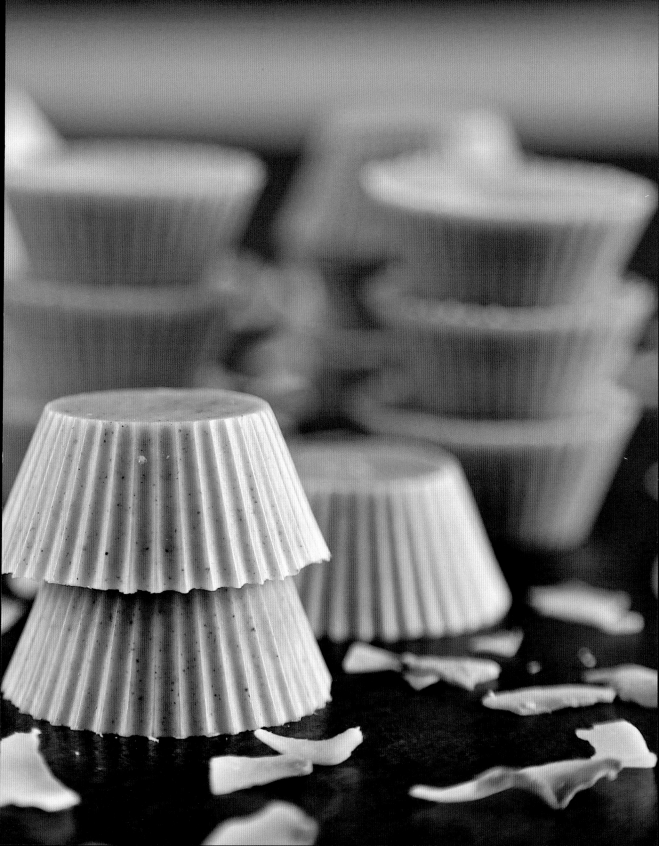

Chewy Hempseed Squares

Hempseeds are low in carbohydrates and high in protein and healthy fats, so they're perfect for making nut-free fat bombs. These sweet, sugar-free squares are bound with homemade condensed milk and framed by thin layers of chocolate.

FOR SQUARES:

1 can (400 ml/13.5 fl oz) coconut milk or equivalent amount of heavy whipping cream

¼ cup (40 g/1.4 oz) erythritol or Swerve, powdered

2 teaspoons sugar-free vanilla extract or 1 teaspoon vanilla powder

1 teaspoon ground cinnamon

¼ cup (55 g/1.9 oz) coconut oil

2 tablespoons (16 g/o.6 oz) ground chia seeds

1 ½ cups (210 g/7.4 oz) hemp seeds, hulled

Few drops liquid stevia, to taste (optional)

FOR COATING:

7.1 ounces (200 g) Homemade Dark Chocolate (page 24)

—

Yield: 16 servings

NUTRITIONAL FACTS

Per serving (1 square): total carbs: 4.4 g; fiber: 2.2 g; net carbs: 2.2 g; protein: 5.8 g; fat: 22.9 g; energy: 231 kcal.

Macronutrient ratio: calories from carbs: 4 percent; protein: 9 percent; fat: 87 percent.

To make the squares: In a small saucepan set over medium heat, bring the coconut milk to a boil. Once simmering, reduce the heat to low. Stir in the erythritol, vanilla, and cinnamon, stirring until the erythritol is dissolved. Cook for 20 to 30 minutes, stirring occasionally, until the milk is creamy and reduced by about half. Remove from the heat and mix in the coconut oil, chia seeds, and hempseeds. If you want a sweeter taste, add the stevia and mix again. Let the mixture sit for 5 to 10 minutes and then refrigerate for about 30 minutes.

To make the coating: Melt the dark chocolate in a double boiler, or heat-proof bowl placed over a small saucepan filled with 1 cup (235 ml) of water, over medium heat. Pour half into an 8 x 8 inch (20 x 20 cm) parchment-lined pan, or a silicone pan. With a spatula, spread the chocolate over the bottom of the pan. Refrigerate for about 15 minutes, or until hardened. Reserve the other half of the melted chocolate for the topping.

Remove both the chocolate and hempseed mixtures from the refrigerator. With a spatula, spread and flatten the hempseed mixture over the chilled chocolate mixture. Top with the remaining melted chocolate. Refrigerate for 45 to 60 minutes to set before slicing. Keep refrigerated for up to 1 week or freeze for up to 3 months.

NOTE:

Nutritional Facts are calculated using Homemade Dark Chocolate made with coconut oil (see recipe on page 24).

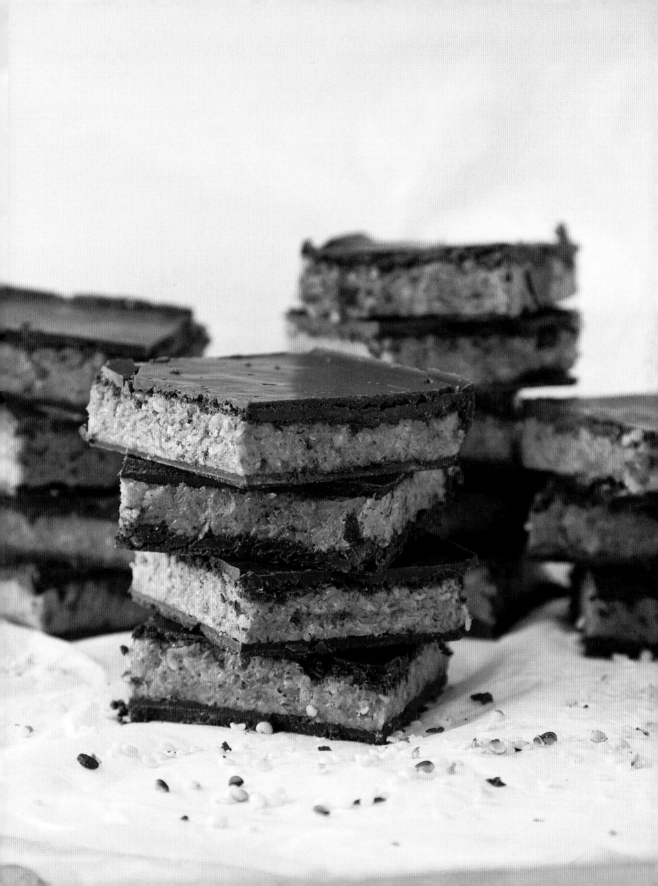

Chocolate-Avocado Truffles

Avocado doesn't turn up in desserts as often as it should because it's high in healthy fats and potassium—and its neutral taste and creamy texture make it a handy tool for creating decadent, low-carb chocolate truffles!

FOR TRUFFLES:

3.5 ounces (100 g) dark chocolate, 90 percent cacao solids or more, or use any of the Homemade Dark Chocolate recipes (page 24)

1 medium (150 g/5.3 oz) avocado, peeled and pitted

¼ cup (60 g/2.1 oz) coconut butter

1 teaspoon sugar-free vanilla extract or ½ teaspoon vanilla powder

½ teaspoon ground cinnamon

Pinch salt

Few drops liquid stevia, to taste (optional)

1 tablespoon (14 g/0.5 oz) macadamia oil or avocado oil, or other light-tasting oil, for shaping the truffles

FOR COATING:

2 tablespoons (10 g/0.4 oz) unsweetened cacao powder, or enough toasted almond flakes, shredded unsweetened coconut, or coconut flakes to cover

—

Yield: 10 servings

To make the truffles: Melt the dark chocolate in a double boiler, or heat-proof bowl placed over a small saucepan filled with 1 cup (235 ml) of water, over medium heat. Remove from heat and set aside.

In a food processor, combine the avocado, coconut butter, vanilla, cinnamon, and salt. Pulse until smooth. With the processor running, slowly drizzle in the melted chocolate. Mix until well combined with the avocado. If you want a sweeter taste, add the stevia. Transfer the mixture to a bowl and refrigerate for about 1 hour, or until solid.

To shape the truffles, dip a spoon or a melon baller in warm water and scoop out ten balls of the chilled mixture. Lightly coat your hands in macadamia oil. Roll the truffles between your palms to form spheres about twice the size of "standard" truffles. Coat them immediately after shaping.

To make the coating: Roll the truffles in your favorite coating. Refrigerate the coated truffles for at least 15 minutes to harden. Keep refrigerated for up to 1 week or freeze for up to 3 months.

NUTRITIONAL FACTS

Per serving (1 truffle): total carbs: 5.3 g; fiber: 3 g; net carbs: 2.3 g; protein: 1.9 g; fat: 12.7 g; energy: 129 kcal.

Macronutrient ratio: calories from carbs: 7 percent; protein: 6 percent; fat: 87 percent.

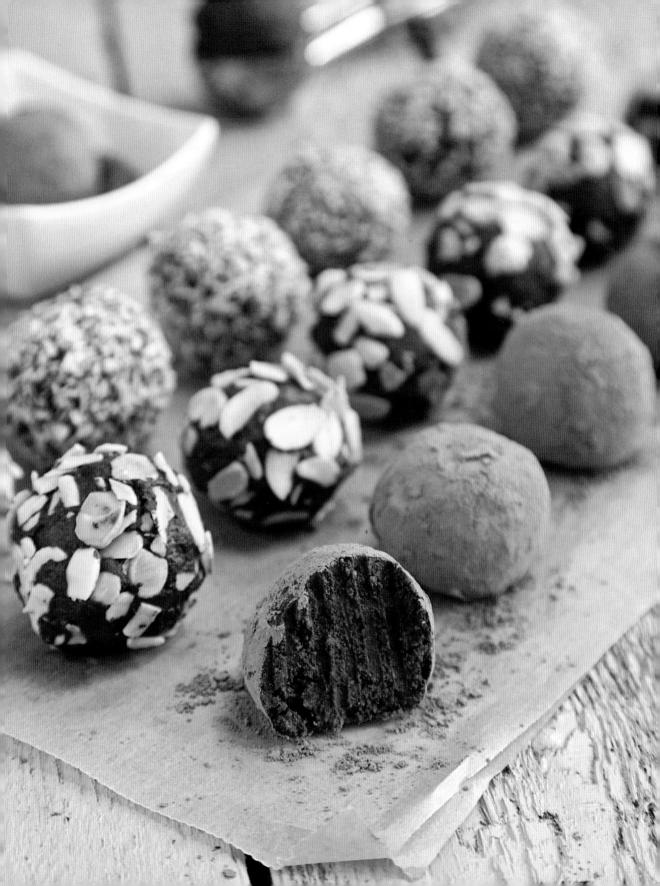

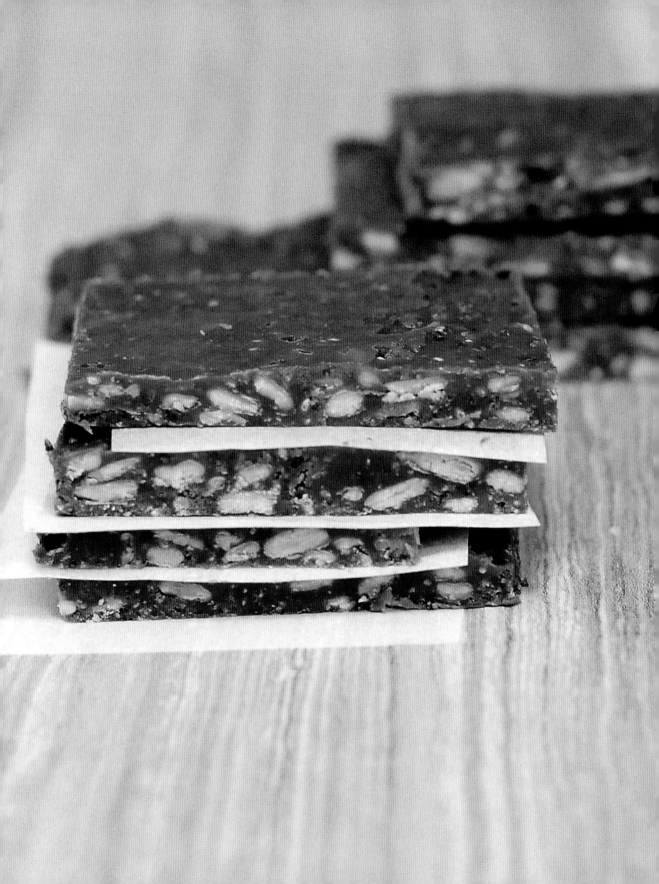

Chocolate Chia Workout Bars

Often referred to as a "superfood" for good reason, chia seeds are a fantastic source of energy for a workout. They digest easily and are absorbed quickly. Just a few bites of these tasty bars will give you a boost of power and keep you sustained for the duration of your activity. Be forewarned: You might not want to eat these too late in the day as the cacao powder might give you too much energy!

1 cup (220 g) coconut butter

⅓ cup (115 g) dark raw honey

½ cup (113 g) salted and roasted sunflower seeds

½ cup (82 g) chia seeds

⅓ cup (27 g) raw cacao powder

¼ cup (20 g) unsweetened shredded coconut

¼ cup (44 g) dark chocolate chips

¼ teaspoon salt

—
Yield: about 12 bars

In a small saucepan over low heat, melt the coconut butter and honey. While that is warming up, in a medium bowl, mix together the sunflower seeds, chia seeds, cacao powder, coconut, chocolate chips, and salt. When the liquids are melted, after about 5 minutes, pour them over the dry ingredients and stir well. Pour the mixture onto a baking sheet lined with parchment paper. Use another piece of parchment paper to flatten the mixture to about ¼ inch (6.5 mm) thick and then refrigerate for 1 hour. Once it has solidified, cut into bars. Store in the fridge or freezer.

NUTRITIONAL FACTS

Per bar: total carbs: 21.9 g; fiber: 5.8 g; net carbs: 15.8 g; protein: 4 g; fat: 21.4 g; calories: 295.

Macronutrient ratio: calories from carbs: 30 percent; protein: 5 percent; fat: 65 percent.

Cinnamon Donut Holes

Donuts are hard to re-create in low-carb form because of the texture and ingredients. Needless to say, these taste like, and have the texture of, a real donut!

½ cup (56 g) coconut flour

2 tablespoons (16 g) psyllium husk powder

¼ cup (48 g) coconut palm sugar, plus 2 tablespoons (24 g) for dipping

¼ teaspoon salt

1 cup (235 ml) water

¼ cup (55 g) grass-fed butter, plus 2 tablespoons (28 g) for dipping (can omit to make dairy-free)

1 tablespoon (7 g) ground cinnamon

—

Yield: About 12 donut holes

NUTRITIONAL FACTS

Per donut: total carbs: 9.5 g; fiber: 3.3 g; net carbs: 6.2 g; protein: 0.7 g; fat: 5.2 g; calories: 85.

Macronutrient ratio: calories from carbs: 44 percent; protein: 3 percent; fat: 53 percent.

Preheat the oven 325°F (170°C, or gas mark 3). Line a baking sheet with parchment paper.

In a medium bowl, mix together the coconut flour, psyllium husk powder, ¼ cup (48 g) coconut palm sugar, and salt. In a small pot, boil the water, turn off stove and then add ¼ cup (55 g) butter and stir until the butter is melted. Add the wet ingredients to the dry. When the mixture has cooled enough for you to handle, squish the dough together until it forms a firm ball.

Tear off golf ball–size pieces of dough and form them into donut holes. Place the balls on the prepared baking sheet. Melt the remaining 2 tablespoons (28 g) butter in a small bowl. In another small bowl, mix together 2 tablespoons (24 g) coconut palm sugar and 1 tablespoon cinnamon. Take each donut hole dough ball and dip it in the butter, making sure to coat it all over. Then, roll it into the sugar-cinnamon mixture. Place it back on the baking sheet and repeat until you have covered all of the balls of dough. Bake about 25 minutes or until a toothpick inserted in the middle comes out clean. Eat them while they are warm!

Alternatively (or in addition to), if you don't want to use cinnamon, you could melt some dark chocolate and drizzle it over the donut holes once they come out of the oven. Mmmmm.

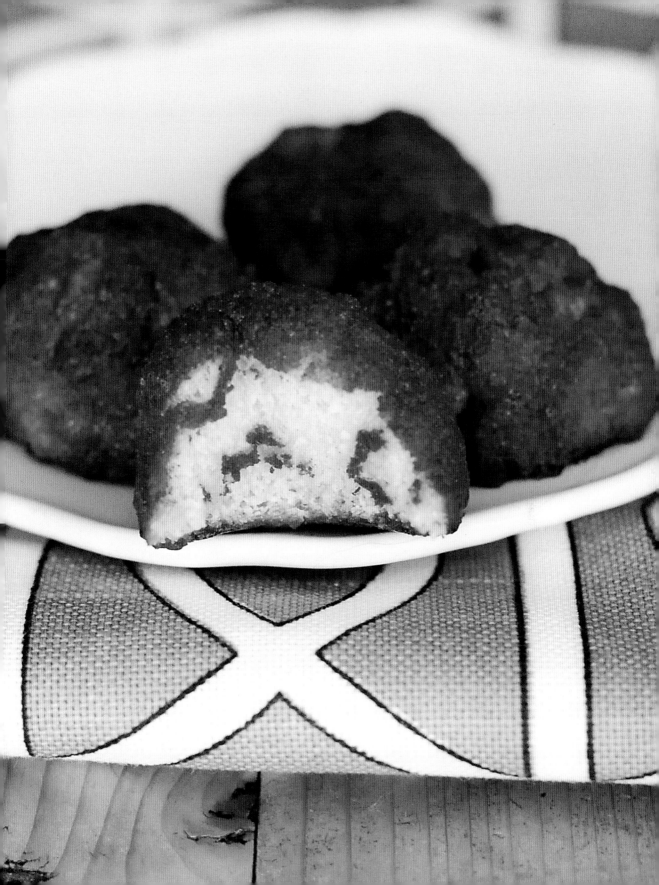

Sweet Bacon Kale

This easy-to-make and supertasty snack is sweet, salty, and so good you'll forget you're eating a superfood.

3 slices nitrate-free bacon, chopped into bite-size pieces

4 big handfuls kale, torn from stems

1 tablespoon (15 ml) apple cider vinegar

¼ teaspoon salt

2 or 3 drops liquid stevia

—

Yield: about 4 servings

In a large skillet over medium heat, cook the bacon until brown and crispy, 8 to 10 minutes. Add the kale and cook for 5 minutes, or until the leaves soften. Mix in the vinegar, salt, and stevia. Serve immediately or save in the fridge for a snack later on.

NUTRITIONAL FACTS

Per serving (1 oz, or 28 g): total carbs: 1.4 g; fiber: 0.6 g; net carbs: 0.8 g; protein: 2.9 g; fat: 3.2 g; calories: 45.

Macronutrient ratio: calories from carbs: 12 percent; protein: 26 percent; fat: 62 percent.

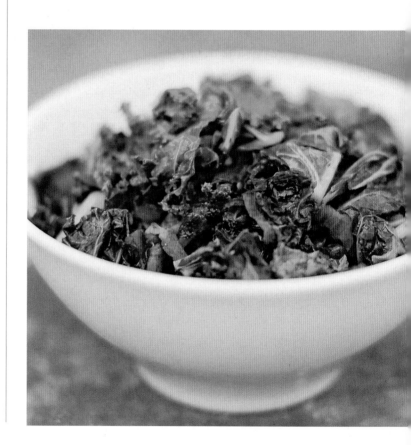

About the Authors

Martina Slajerova is a health and food blogger living in the United Kingdom. She holds a degree in economics and worked in auditing, but has always been passionate about nutrition and healthy living. Martina loves food, science, photography, and creating new recipes. She is a firm believer in low-carb living and regular exercise. As a science geek, she bases her views on valid research and has firsthand experience of what it means to be on a low-carb diet. Both are reflected on her blog, in her KetoDiet apps, and this book.

The KetoDiet is an ongoing project she started with her partner in 2012 and includes *The KetoDiet Cookbook, Fat Bombs*, and the KetoDiet apps for the iPad and iPhone (www.ketodietapp.com). When creating recipes, she doesn't focus on just the carb content: You won't find any processed foods, unhealthy vegetable oils, or artificial sweeteners in her recipes.

This book and the KetoDiet apps are for people who follow a healthy low-carb lifestyle. Martina's mission is to help you reach your goals, whether it's your dream weight or simply eating healthy food. You can find even more low-carb recipes, diet plans, and information about the keto diet on her blog: www.ketodietapp.com/blog.

Landria Voigt, C.H.H.C., is a nutritional consultant and public speaker. In her twenties, she was diagnosed with an autoimmune disease and for years struggled to keep flares in check with traditional, conventional approaches. After more than a decade of suffering and frustration, she took her health into her own hands, casting aside the drugs and carefully experimenting with her own diet. The results were nothing short of miraculous.

As a result of her journey, she came to appreciate the power of nutrition and how challenging it can be to separate facts from dubious marketing spin when choosing the right foods for one's self and family. Now she is on a mission to help others enjoy healthier living through informed eating. Through public speaking engagements and consulting at The Atlanta Center for Holistic and Integrative Medicine for Taz "Dr. Taz" Bhatia, M.D., patients in Atlanta, she shares her knowledge and most up-to-date research on the ever changing subjects of food and wellness.

Through her blog stiritup.me, Landria shares her healthy recipes aimed at pleasing even the most finicky of palates, as well as forward-thinking ideas about nutrition.

Continued

In retrospect, **Dana Carpender's** career seems inevitable: She's been cooking since she had to stand on a step stool to reach the stove. She was also a dangerously sugar-addicted child, eventually stealing from her parents to support her habit, and was in Weight Watchers by age eleven. At nineteen, Dana read her first book on nutrition and recognized herself in a list of symptoms of reactive hypoglycemia. She ditched sugar and white flour, and was dazzled by the near-instantaneous improvement in her physical and mental health. A lifetime nutrition buff was born.

Unfortunately, in the late eighties and early nineties, Dana got sucked into low-fat/high-carb mania, and whole-grain-and-beaned her way up to a size 20, with nasty energy swings, constant hunger, and borderline high blood pressure. In 1995, she read a nutrition book from the 1950s that stated that obesity had nothing to do with how much one ate, but was rather a carbohydrate intolerance disease. She thought, "What the heck, might as well give it a try." Three days later, her clothes were loose, her hunger was gone, and her energy level was through the roof. She never looked back, and has now been low carb for nineteen years and counting—a third of her life.

Realizing that this change was permanent, and being a cook at heart, Dana set about creating as varied and satisfying a cuisine as she could with a minimal carb load. And being an enthusiastic, gregarious sort, she started sharing her experience. By 1997 she was writing about it. The upshot is more than 2,500 recipes published, and over a million books sold—and she still has ideas left to try!

Dana lives in Bloomington, Indiana, with her husband, three dogs, and a cat, all of whom are well and healthily fed.

Index

Almond and Cashew Butter, 10
Almond Bliss Bars, 89
Almond Bliss Butter
  Almond Bliss Smoothie, 108
  recipe, 22
Almond butter
  Blonde Snack Bars, 86
  Chocolate Chip Muffins, 77
  Cinnamon Raisin Bars, 80
  Pumpkin Bars, 82
  Supersmart Bars, 49
Almond flour/meal
  Chocolate Chip Cookie Butter, 18
  Chocolate Chip Muffins, 77
  Favorite Crackers, 78
  Italian Meatballs, 35
  Mini Zucchini Muffins, 74
  N'Oatmeal Cookies, 66
  Savory Baked Chicken Nuggets, 30
Almond milk
  Almond Bliss Smoothie, 108
  Creamy Dark Hot Chocolate, 93
  Creamy White Hot Chocolate, 94
Almonds
  Almond and Cashew Butter, 10
  Almond Bliss Bars, 89
  Almond Bliss Butter, 22
  Berry Nut Butter, 15
  Chocolate-Hazelnut Butter, 12
  Crispy Maple Granola, 73
  Kale Salad, 54
  N'Oatmeal Cookies, 66
Arrowroot powder, in N'Oatmeal
Cookies, 66
Asparagus, Prosciutto-Wrapped, 60
Avocado
  Bacon and Guacamole Fat Bombs,
  118
  Chocolate-Avocado Truffles, 132
  Chorizo and Avocado Fat Bombs,
  42
  Green Deviled Eggs & Bacon, 58
  Key Lime Smoothie, 107

Bacon
  Bacon and Guacamole Fat Bombs,
  118
  Bacon & Egg Maple Muffins, 44
  Green Deviled Eggs & Bacon, 58

Pork Belly Fat Bombs, 64
  Sweet Bacon Kale, 138
Bars
  Almond Bliss Bars, 89
  Blonde Snack Bars, 86
  Chocolate Chia Workout Bars, 135
  Cinnamon Raisin Bars, 80
  Pumpkin Bars, 82
Basil (fresh)
  Ham and Cheese Fat Bombs, 121
  Herbed Cheese Fat Bombs, 38
  Sun-Dried Tomato Chicken Sliders,
  32
Beef (ground), in Italian Meatballs, 35
Berry powder, in Berry Nut Butter, 15
Blonde Snack Bars, 86
Blue cheese
  Stilton and Chive Fat Bombs, 117
  Waldorf Salad Fat Bombs, 53
Brussels sprouts
  Kale Salad, 54
  Zesty Walnut Brussels Sprouts, 57

Cacao butter
  Almond Bliss Butter, 22
  Homemade Dark Chocolate, 24–25
  Homemade White Chocolate, 27
  White Chocolate and Macadamia
  Butter, 15
Cacao nibs, in Earl Grey Truffles, 126
Cacao powder
  Chocolate Chia Workout Bars, 135
  Chocolate-Hazelnut Butter, 12
  Homemade Dark Chocolate, 24–25
Cardamom pods, in Creamy Dark Hot
Chocolate, 93
Cashew flour, in Savory Baked
Chicken Nuggets, 30
Cashews
  Almond and Cashew Butter, 10
  Supersmart Bars, 49
Cauliflower
  Cauliflower Hummus, 61
  Cauliflower Pizza Bites, 36
Cheddar cheese, in Ham and Cheese
Fat Bombs, 121
Chewy Hempseed Squares, 130
Chia seeds
  Almond Bliss Smoothie, 108

Chewy Hempseed Squares, 130
  Chocolate Chia Workout Bars, 135
  Crispy Maple Granola, 73
  Favorite Crackers, 78
Chicken
  Savory Baked Chicken Nuggets, 30
  Sun-Dried Tomato Chicken Sliders,
  32
Chile-Lime Peanuts, 81
Chives (fresh)
  Chorizo and Avocado Fat Bombs,
  42
  Smoked Mackerel Pâté Fat Bombs,
  125
  Stilton and Chive Fat Bombs, 117
  Waldorf Salad Fat Bombs, 53
Chocolate-Avocado Truffles, 132
Chocolate Chia Workout Bars, 135
Chocolate Chip Cookie Butter, 18
Chocolate Chip Muffins, 77
Chocolate chips. See Dark chocolate
chips
Chocolate-Hazelnut Butter, 12
Chocolate, unsweetened
  Creamy Dark Hot Chocolate, 93
  Earl Grey Truffles, 126
  Homemade Dark Chocolate, 24–25
Chorizo sausage, in Chorizo and
Avocado Fat Bombs, 42
Cinnamon Donut Holes, 136
Cococcino, 98
Coconut (unsweetened shredded), 73
  Almond Bliss Bars, 89
  Almond Bliss Butter, 22
  Almond Bliss Smoothie, 108
  Chocolate Chia Workout Bars, 135
  Coconut and Pecan Butter, 11
  Pistachio-Coconut Butter, 20
  Supersmart Bars, 49
  Toasted Coconut Cups, 128
Coconut and Pecan Butter, 11
Coconut butter
  Berry Nut Butter, 15
  Chocolate-Avocado Truffles, 132
  Chocolate Chia Workout Bars, 135
  White Chocolate and Macadamia
  Butter, 15
Coconut Chai, 99

Coconut flour
  Bacon & Egg Maple Muffins, 44
  Chocolate Chia Workout Bars, 136
  Cinnamon Donut Holes, 136
  Flatbread "PB&J," 63
  Pumpkin Bars, 82
  Pumpkin Chocolate Chip Muffins, 46
Coconut milk
  Almond Bliss Smoothie, 108
  Bacon & Egg Maple Muffins, 44
  Chewy Hempseed Squares, 130
  Cococcino, 98
  Coconut Chai, 99
  Coconut-Vanilla Coffee, 98
  Creamy Dark Hot Chocolate, 93
  Creamy Keto Coffee, 97
  Creamy White Hot Chocolate, 94
  Earl Grey Truffles, 126
  Pumpkin Chocolate Chip Muffins, 46
  Vanilla-Keto Ice Cream, 69
Coconut milk powder, in Homemade White Chocolate, 27
Coconut nectar, in Supersmart Bars, 49
Coconut oil
  Almond Bliss Bars, 89
  Berry Nut Butter, 15
  Chewy Hempseed Squares, 130
  Chile-Lime Peanuts, 81
  Chocolate Chip Cookie Butter, 18
  Chocolate Chip Muffins, 77
  Creamy Keto Coffee, 97
  Flatbread "PB&J," 63
  Homemade Dark Chocolate, 24–25
  Pumpkin Chocolate Chip Muffins, 46
  Supersmart Bars, 49
  Toasted Coconut Cups, 128
  Zesty Walnut Brussels Sprouts, 57
Coconut palm sugar
  Blonde Snack Bars, 86
  Chocolate Chia Workout Bars, 136
  Chocolate Chip Muffins, 77
  Cinnamon Raisin Bars, 80
  Mini Zucchini Muffins, 74
  N'Oatmeal Cookies, 66
  "Peanut Butter" Cookies, 84
  Pumpkin Bars, 82
  Pumpkin Chocolate Chip Muffins, 46

Coconut-Vanilla Coffee, 98
Coffee
  Coconut-Vanilla Coffee, 98
  Creamy Keto Coffee, 97
Cookies
  N'Oatmeal Cookies, 66
  "Peanut Butter" Cookies, 84
Crackers, Favorite, 78
Cranberries (dried), in Kale Salad, 54
Cream cheese
  Ham and Cheese Fat Bombs, 121
  Herbed Cheese Fat Bombs, 38
  Pepperoni Pizza Fat Bombs, 114
  Salmon Pâté Fat Bombs, 40
  Stilton and Chive Fat Bombs, 117
  Veggie and Cheese Fat Bombs, 122
  Waldorf Salad Fat Bombs, 53
Creamed coconut milk
  Almond Bliss Bars, 89
  Creamy Orange Smoothie, 104
  Fat-Burning Vanilla Smoothie, 100
  Key Lime Smoothie, 107
  Raspberry and Vanilla Smoothie, 103
  Vanilla-Keto Ice Cream, 69
Creamy Dark Hot Chocolate, 93
Creamy Keto Coffee, 97
Creamy Orange Smoothie, 104
Crispy Maple Granola, 73
Crispy Okra Sticks, 113
Cucumber, in Smoked Mackerel Pâté Fat Bombs, 125
Currants
  Cinnamon Raisin Bars, 80
  Mini Zucchini Muffins, 74

Dark chocolate. *See also* Homemade Dark Chocolate
  Almond Bliss Butter, 22
  Chocolate-Avocado Truffles, 132
  Chocolate-Hazelnut Butter, 12
Dark chocolate chips
  Blonde Snack Bars, 86
  Chocolate Chia Workout Bars, 135
  Chocolate Chip Cookie Butter, 18
  Chocolate Chip Muffins, 77
  Pumpkin Chocolate Chip Muffins, 46
  Supersmart Bars, 49
Deviled Eggs & Bacon, 58
Dill (fresh), in Salmon Pâté Fat

Bombs, 40
Dip, Roasted Red Pepper, 62
Donut Holes, Cinnamon, 136

Earl Grey Truffles, 126
Eggnog-Macadamia Butter, 14
Eggs
  Bacon & Egg Maple Muffins, 44
  Blonde Snack Bars, 86
  Chocolate Chip Muffins, 77
  Cinnamon Raisin Bars, 80
  Green Deviled Eggs & Bacon, 58
  hardboiled, in Chorizo and Avocado Fat Bombs, 42
  Italian Meatballs, 35
  Mini Zucchini Muffins, 74
  N'Oatmeal Cookies, 66
  Pumpkin Bars, 82
  Pumpkin Chocolate Chip Muffins, 46
  Vanilla-Keto Ice Cream, 69
Egg yolks
  Chocolate Chip Cookie Butter, 18
  Creamy Keto Coffee, 97
  Creamy Orange Smoothie, 104
  Fat-Burning Vanilla Smoothie, 100
  Vanilla-Keto Ice Cream, 69
Espresso, in Cococcino, 98

Fat bombs
  Chorizo and Avocado Fat Bombs, 42
  Ham and Cheese Fat Bombs, 121
  Herbed Cheese Fat Bombs, 38
  Pepperoni Pizza Fat Bombs, 114
  Pork Belly Fat Bombs, 64
  Salmon Pâté Fat Bombs, 40
  Smoked Mackerel Pâté Fat Bombs, 125
  Stilton and Chive Fat Bombs, 117
  Veggie and Cheese Fat Bombs, 122
  Waldorf Salad Fat Bombs, 53
Fat-Burning Vanilla Smoothie, 100
Favorite Crackers, 78
Flatbread "PB&J," 63
Flaxseed meal
  Favorite Crackers, 78
  Mini Zucchini Muffins, 74
Food extracts, for fat bombs, 16

Glycerin, 16

Goat cheese
    Cauliflower Pizza Bites, 36
    Veggie and Cheese Fat Bombs, 122
Gouda cheese, in Ham and Cheese
Fat Bombs, 121
Granola, Crispy Maple, 73
Green Deviled Eggs & Bacon, 58
Ground beef, in Italian Meatballs, 35

Ham and Cheese Fat Bombs, 121
Hazelnuts, in Chocolate-Hazelnut
Butter, 12
Heavy whipping cream
    Almond Bliss Smoothie, 108
    Chewy Hempseed Squares, 130
    Creamy Dark Hot Chocolate, 93
    Creamy Keto Coffee, 97
    Creamy White Hot Chocolate, 94
    Earl Grey Truffles, 126
    Key Lime Smoothie, 107
Hemp seeds, in Chewy Hempseed
Squares, 130
Herbs (fresh). *See also* Basil (fresh);
Chives (fresh); Parsley (fresh)
    Herbed Cheese Fat Bombs, 38
    Pepperoni Pizza Fat Bombs, 114
Homemade Dark Chocolate
    Almond Bliss Bar, 89
    Chewy Hempseed Squares, 130
    Chocolate-Avocado Truffles, 132
    Chocolate Chip Cookie Butter, 18
    recipe, 24–25
Homemade White Chocolate
    Creamy White Hot Chocolate, 94
    Earl Grey Truffles, 126
    recipe, 27
Honey, in Chocolate Chia Workout
Bars, 135
Horseradish, in Pork Belly Fat Bombs,
64
Hot chocolate
    Creamy Dark Hot Chocolate, 93
    Creamy White Hot Chocolate, 94
Hummus, Cauliflower, 61

Ice Cream, Vanilla-Keto, 69
Italian Meatballs, 35
Italian seasoning, in Favorite Crackers,
78

Kale
    Kale Salad, 54
    Sweet Bacon Kale, 138
Key Lime Smoothie, 107

Lettuce leaves
    Pork Belly Fat Bombs, 64
    Salmon Pâté Fat Bombs, 40
Lime juice
    Bacon and Guacamole Fat Bombs,
    118
    Chile-Lime Peanuts, 81
    Green Deviled Eggs & Bacon, 58
    Key Lime Smoothie, 107

Macadamia nuts
    Berry Nut Butter, 15
    Chocolate-Hazelnut Butter, 12
    Eggnog-Macadamia Butter, 14
    Pistachio-Coconut Butter, 20
    White Chocolate and Macadamia
    Butter, 15
Mackerel fillet, in Smoked Mackerel
Pâté Fat Bombs, 125
Maple extract, in Spiced Maple and
Pecan Butter, 16
Maple syrup
    Bacon & Egg Maple Muffins, 44
    Cinnamon Raisin Bars, 80
    Crispy Maple Granola, 73
    N'Oatmeal Cookies, 66
    Pumpkin Bars, 82
    Pumpkin Chocolate Chip Muffins,
    46
    Sweet & Spicy Spiced Pepitas, 113
Mascarpone cheese
    Creamy Orange Smoothie, 104
    Fat-Burning Vanilla Smoothie, 100
    Raspberry and Vanilla Smoothie,
    103
Meatballs, Italian, 35
Mozzarella cheese
    Cauliflower Pizza Bites, 36
    Pepperoni Pizza Fat Bombs, 114
Muffins
    Bacon & Egg Maple Muffins, 44
    Chocolate Chip Muffins, 77
    Mini Zucchini Muffins, 74
    Pumpkin Chocolate Chip Muffins,
    46

Mushrooms, in Veggie and Cheese Fat
Bombs, 122

N'Oatmeal Cookies, 66
Nut butters. *See also* Almond butter
    Almond and Cashew Butter, 10
    Almond Bliss Butter, 22
    Berry Nut Butter, 15
    Chocolate-Hazelnut Butter, 12
    Coconut and Pecan Butter, 11
    Eggnog-Macadamia Butter, 14
    Pistachio-Coconut Butter, 20
    Spiced Maple and Pecan Butter, 16
    White Chocolate and Macadamia
    Butter, 15

Okra, in Crispy Okra Sticks, 113
Olives
    Ham and Cheese Fat Bombs, 121
    Herbed Cheese Fat Bombs, 38
Orange Smoothie, Creamy, 104

Pancetta, in Pork Belly Fat Bombs, 64
Parma ham, in Ham and Cheese Fat
Bombs, 121
Parmesan cheese
    Cauliflower Pizza Bites, 36
    Herbed Cheese Fat Bombs, 38
    Kale Salad, 54
    Pepperoni Pizza Fat Bombs, 114
Parsley (fresh)
    Italian Meatballs, 35
    Stilton and Chive Fat Bombs, 117
"Peanut Butter" Cookies, 84
Peanut Hummus, 61
Peanuts, Chile-Lime, 81
Pecans
    Coconut and Pecan Butter, 11
    Crispy Maple Granola, 73
    N'Oatmeal Cookies, 66
    Spiced Maple and Pecan Butter, 16
    Waldorf Salad Fat Bombs, 53
Pepitas, in Sweet & Spicy Spiced
Pepitas, 113
Pepperoni Pizza Fat Bombs, 114
Pistachio nuts, in Pistachio-Coconut
Butter, 20
Pizza Bites, Cauliflower, 36
Pizza sauce, in Cauliflower Pizza
Bites, 36

Pork
  Ham and Cheese Fat Bombs, 121
  Pork Belly Fat Bombs, 64
  Prosciutto-Wrapped Asparagus, 60
Prosciutto-Wrapped Asparagus, 60
Psyllium husk powder
  Chocolate Chia Workout Bars, 136
  Cinnamon Donut Holes, 136
  Flatbread "PB&J," 63
Pumpkin pie spice
  Pumpkin Bars, 82
  Pumpkin Chocolate Chip Muffins, 46
  Sweet & Spicy Spiced Pepitas, 113
Pumpkin purée
  Pumpkin Bars, 82
  Pumpkin Chocolate Chip Muffins, 46
Pumpkin seeds, in Pumpkin Sun Butter, 21

Raisins
  Cinnamon Raisin Bars, 80
  Mini Zucchini Muffins, 74
  N'Oatmeal Cookies, 66
Raspberries, in Raspberry and Vanilla Smoothie, 103
Roasted red peppers, in Roasted Red Pepper Dip, 62
Rum extract, in Eggnog-Macadamia Butter, 14

Salad, Kale, 54
Salmon (smoked), in Salmon Pâté Fat Bombs, 40
Salmon Pâté Fat Bombs, 40
Sausage
  Chorizo and Avocado Fat Bombs, 42
  Italian Meatballs, 35

Savory Baked Chicken Nuggets, 30
Sesame seeds, in Savory Baked Chicken Nuggets, 30
Smoked Mackerel Pâté Fat Bombs, 125
Smoked salmon, in Salmon Pâté Fat Bombs, 40
Smoothies
  Almond Bliss Smoothie, 108
  Creamy Orange Smoothie, 104
  Fat-Burning Vanilla Smoothie, 100
  Key Lime Smoothie, 107
  Raspberry and Vanilla Smoothie, 103
Spiced Maple and Pecan Butter, 16
Spinach, in Veggie and Cheese Fat Bombs, 122
Stilton and Chive Fat Bombs, 117
Strawberries, in Flatbread "PB&J," 63
Sun-Dried Tomato Chicken Sliders, 32
Sundried tomatoes
  Herbed Cheese Fat Bombs, 38
  Sun-Dried Tomato Chicken Sliders, 32
Sunflower seed butter
  Cinnamon Raisin Bars, 80
  Flatbread "PB&J," 63
  "Peanut Butter" Cookies, 84
Sunflower seeds
  Chocolate Chia Workout Bars, 135
  Pumpkin Sun Butter, 21
Supersmart Bars, 49
Sweet Bacon Kale, 138
Sweet & Spicy Spiced Pepitas, 113
Swerve. See Erythritol or Swerve

Tahini, in Cauliflower Hummus, 61
Tea
  Coconut Chai, 99
  Earl Grey Truffles, 126

Toasted Coconut Cups, 128
Tomato sauce, in Cauliflower Pizza Bites, 36
Truffles
  Chocolate-Avocado Truffles, 132
  Earl Grey Truffles, 126

Unsweetened chocolate. See Chocolate, unsweetened

Vanilla-Keto Ice Cream, 69
Veggie and Cheese Fat Bombs, 122

Waldorf Salad Fat Bombs, 53
Walnuts
  Cinnamon Raisin Bars, 80
  Crispy Maple Granola, 73
  Mini Zucchini Muffins, 74
  N'Oatmeal Cookies, 66
  Pumpkin Bars, 82
  Roasted Red Pepper Dip, 62
  Supersmart Bars, 49
  Waldorf Salad Fat Bombs, 53
  Zesty Walnut Brussels Sprouts, 57
Whipped cream. See also Heavy whipping cream
  Almond Bliss Smoothie, 108
  Creamy Orange Smoothie, 104
  Fat-Burning Vanilla Smoothie, 100
  Key Lime Smoothie, 107
  Raspberry and Vanilla Smoothie, 103
White Chocolate and Macadamia Butter, 15

Zesty Walnut Brussels Sprouts, 57
Zucchini, in Mini Zucchini Muffins, 74